A Healthy Approach
German Cancer Clinic

My personal story of triumph over breast cancer!

Laura L Jackson RN
www.ahealthyapproach.com

ISBN:1490358668
ISBN-13:9781490358666

DEDICATION

I want to dedicate this journal to my Lord and Savior, Jesus Christ. You are faithful and true to your word. We prayed for your guidance and you truly opened and closed the various doors of treatment options to keep us walking on your path to healing. Thank you for the relationships we made, experiences we had, and your comforting presence throughout my journey. Miracles do happen!

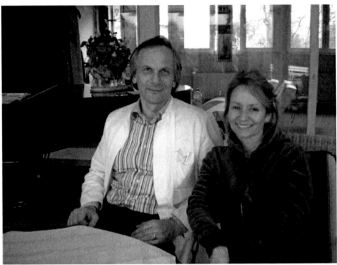

Dr. Alexander Herzog, M.D. and me, Laura Jackson
at his German Cancer Klinik (Clinic)

ACKNOWLEDGEMENTS

Aunt Mary, Aunt Frances, Grandma Jeanne, Pastor Tom and his wife Carol, and Janice, I want to thank you for your support. I will be forever grateful to you, who gave of your time and energy, away from your own families, to come live in my home and care for my 3 children, granddad, and pets (a dog, 2 cats and a fish) while Chuck and I traveled to Germany.

Thank you to all those who were there to support and help me and my family through this trial. Without you, none of this would have been possible. Thank you to all my neighbors, friends, school family and church family for the dinners and words of comfort. Diane S., tell the girls, Lilly and Amanda, they are very smart and I so thank them for taking care of my little Evan, making sure he gets to school safely each day!!! They're showing great responsibility and a caring attitude for such young ladies!

Thank you to all who responded to my journal entries which made me feel loved and helped me get through my "homesickness" which occurred on a daily basis. Traveling to a foreign country was a fearful endeavor for me as a nurse working in a huge healthcare system in Florida. I must also give thanks to the wonderful nurses (Krankenswelters) at the German clinic (klinik) for their kindness and compassion as they guided me through each day in a caring and professional manner. The cafeteria ladies, massage therapists, and one very special housekeeper, had lots of smiles, hugs and words of encouragement whenever I needed them.

It was such a comfort to see their familiar smiling faces upon each return trip to the klinik for the duration of my treatments. They all knew how to make me laugh too. I sure needed that!

Special thanks to my husband, Chuck, and my sister, Clarissa, for reminding me daily of God's peace and healing power, through each fearful day, and their endless positive outlook and daily, constant words of comfort and encouragement.

I want to thank Granddad and my children, Morgan, Tyler, and Evan, for adapting through all the changes and disruptions in our home, and remaining cheerful and positive as different people cared for them.

Finally, I want to express my utmost gratitude and respect for Dr. Herzog. You are the definition of A Healthy Approach to treating cancer. Thank you so much for your skill, support, and encouragement. You are, without a doubt, a great integrative oncologist!

CONTENTS

INTRODUCTION

This book is intended to give a first-hand look at what I went through with my treatments, feelings, and progress, but also what it was like traveling to a foreign country for medical treatment. I wanted to provide information on the "what", "how" and "why" of the particular German cancer therapies that I received. I would have loved to read, ahead of time, about what awaited me as we headed out of our native country to unfamiliar ground for medical treatment.

Being an RN health educator for years, I wanted to explain all my experiences in receiving treatment in a foreign country in order to help others who may be interested in stepping "outside the box" of traditional therapy, and pursue a less toxic, and in my opinion, a more effective, healthier approach.

This is my story, now available in a fun, easy to read format, which also explains each treatment I received and why I was receiving it. It's written from a patient's viewpoint so that anyone can understand the information, as well as appreciate the journey.

I call it "A Healthy Approach" because my husband, Chuck, and I spent weeks researching a better way to fight cancer without resorting to destroying my body in the meantime. Although we would rather not have to travel to Germany to find the treatment we were looking for, travel to Germany we did!

January 2, 2009, I was diagnosed with stage III adenocarcinoma breast cancer. Just a short 4 months later on May 22, 2009, I was diagnosed as "Cancer Free" and "In Total Remission" by my German oncologist, verified by my radiologist and doctor here in the US.

Yes, you read right! Within a four month period of time I went from receiving the most horrifying news in my life, to having one of the most unbelievable days in my life. Did I mention I beat breast cancer without any surgery except one lymph node for diagnosis, had no radiation, and just a very small amount of chemotherapy. Well I did! Praise God, I did!

Even though my treatment options may not be the best approach for you, from a nurse's standpoint, I encourage you to explore other options outside of the standard point of care that fails so many times.

One day while working in the hospital and assisting a doctor as he was seeing one of his patients, I had an epiphany, a turning point or new understanding, of the medical system. This was very early on in my career, about 5 years in. The doctor came in like a whirlwind, spoke to the patient using medical jargon, scribbled on a notepad, tapped the patient on the ankle a couple of times, more in a friendly way than anything medical (this was a heart patient), then the doctor left as quickly as he arrived, as he looked at me and pointed toward the patient. I knew this meant for me to explain all that was just said. The visit was about 5 or 10 minutes, at most. The patient was left looking at me with a confused look. I explained what the doctor told him in terms he could understand and even made an excuse for the doctor's visit being so short. But as I was watching the doctor speak to my patient and seeing that he wasn't really understanding what the doctor was saying, it hit me like a brick wall, "doctors don't take care of people, people have to take care of themselves", as in, taking charge of your own health. The majority of doctors don't have the time to sit down with every patient and tell them what they should eat, how much to exercise, how to get over bad habits and develop good ones, and then be there to make sure his or her patient obeys. Nor can they take a person who has abused their health for years and in a 10 minute office or hospital visit, fix everything!

My advice is to do research and be well informed about good health, with your own thoughts and questions. Understand everything that's going on with your own care, or have someone with you who can do this for you. Don't be afraid to do your own research if "something doesn't seem right". After all, doctors are humans too, and most of them seem to be in such a hurry! Keep in mind, not all doctors are like this, but it's not uncommon.

Currently, I have a website called AHealthyApproach.com where I post common sense ideas and suggestions on keeping healthy naturally, with special emphasis on remaining cancer free. You can also email me with questions about my German treatments at LauraRn@AHealthyApproach.com.

Whatever you decide, I want to express that there is a whole world of alternative treatments that need to be explored. The internet is a wonderful thing. I don't believe that any one treatment is best for everyone, but for me, a combination of foods, supplements, detoxing, and managing stress, in addition to finding a treatment that you're comfortable with, is a great place to start.

DISCLAIMER

Laura Jackson is not a doctor. The entire contents of this book are based upon the opinions and experiences of Laura. The information in this book is not intended to replace a one-on-one relationship with a qualified health care professional and is not intended as medical advice. Nothing herein is intended to diagnose, treat, cure or prevent any disease. This book is a sharing of knowledge and information from the research and experience of Laura only, and should not be construed as medical advice. In no way should anyone infer that Laura is practicing medicine. Laura assumes no responsibility for inaccuracies in any of her source materials or statements, nor does she assume responsibility for how this material is used. This book is in no way comprehensive and Laura encourages you to make your own health care and nutrition decisions based upon your research and in partnership with a qualified health care professional. Laura's statements regarding any treatments for cancer have not been evaluated by the FDA.

JOURNAL ENTRY

SURPRISE, SURPRISE! (and not in a good way)

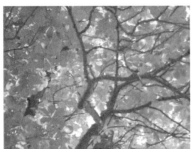

My name is Laura Jackson. I have been a Registered Nurse (RN) since 1985 and work as a healthcare educator for a major hospital system in central Florida. I am married with three children; one daughter and 2 sons. I have always exercised pretty regularly, eaten healthy, or so I thought, and had regular mammograms. Just before Thanksgiving, 2008, I discovered a lump under my arm. It turned out to be a swollen lymph node which I had removed in December for testing. On January 2, 2009 my husband and I were told that breast cancer cells were found in the removed lymph node. Shortly after that the breast surgeon diagnosed me with stage III adenocarcinoma breast cancer. This came to us as an absolute shock as I was only 44 and felt I was in very good physical shape, although I was a little overweight.

From the beginning, I was against the concept of radiation and chemotherapy. My husband and I both have lost parents and relatives to cancer. They all followed the traditional route of surgery, radiation and chemotherapy.

We feel that the radiation and chemo treatments heavily damage the body's ability to fight off cancer, especially if it were to reoccur in the future. It also seems that if the cancer does come back, it's usually very chemo resistant and comes back with a vengeance. This is what happened to our loved ones.

Our experience, along with my medical knowledge, has led us to look for alternatives to standard U.S. treatment protocols.

Through hours upon hours of research and prayer, we made the decision to seek treatment from Dr. Alexander Herzog's Integrative Cancer Clinic in Germany. I also had a local physician at home for follow-up care, MRI scans, and any other assistance needed upon our return.

Why Are We Seeking Treatment In Germany?

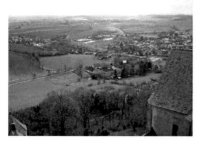

The first question we always get is "Why Germany?". The cancer treatment philosophy in Germany is very different then the philosophy in the U.S. I compare it to treating the whole forest instead of just the tree. We felt the traditional view of cancer in the U.S. is that the cancer (the tree) is the disease and the focus is on killing, or shrinking, the cancer to cure the patient.

Whereas the German view seems to be that the cancer is a symptom of a greater problem within the patient's body (the forest). This view not only focuses on killing the cancer, but also includes treating the body, through various therapies and detoxing programs designed to protect and support the body's healthy cells before, during, and after treatment.

In other words, the patient is not really cured until the body is in a condition to be able to fight off any future cancer reoccurrences. After all, the typical healthy body is killing cancer cells that develop in it every day. That's right; your body is killing cancer cells every day! When your body, for whatever reason, can't kill as many cancer cells as are being created, you are on your way to developing a cancer tumor.

Another reason we chose Germany is because there are several therapies and medications, such as hyperthermia and Iscador that are in clinical trials in the U.S. (unavailable to me) but are standard treatment protocols in Germany. I will post the details of the different treatments I will be receiving in this journal.

A Bright Future.

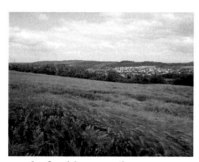

I believe that everyone faces trials in life. Sometimes the trial may seem bigger than life, bigger than we can handle. However, with God on your side, you can handle anything!

I prayed that the Lord bring healing, strength, comfort, and guidance throughout this trial, and that this experience would somehow be used to help others in need of guidance and answers.

MY JOURNEY BEGINS

FIRST TRIP TO GERMANY

Thursday, February 5, 2009 6:42 PM

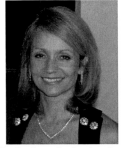

BIG PLANS AHEAD!

Next week, Friday the 13th of all days, Chuck and I fly to Germany. I will be receiving treatments to rid my body of breast cancer cells, which were also found in my lymph nodes.

The clinic, which has a great reputation, is located in Bad Salzhausen, meaning "bath salt house", just outside Frankfurt. From what I understand, my three weeks of treatments will include whole body detox, nutritional, and enzyme programs to supercharge my immune system. It will also include hyperthermia treatments, Iscador medication, physical therapy, and possibly low-dose chemo to get rid of any cancer. There will probably be other therapies too. We won't know until I have had a checkup by the German physicians after we check in at the klinik (in Germany it's spelled klinik)

Again, Chuck and I want to give a HUGE thanks to all those who have helped us out with dinners, moral support, and prayers during this difficult time in our lives. While in Germany we would like to welcome any words of encouragement from you on my journal website. Each evening we will look forward to reading the messages.

Friday, February 13, 2009 10:41 AM

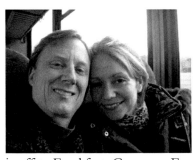

On Our Way to "Out of My Comfort Zone"

Well, it's been wild and crazy with packing and making sure we have our passports and lots of warm clothing. It's extremely cold right now in Germany so we had to borrow several snowy outfits, but we are on our way to the airport. First stop is Cincinnati for a three hour layover. Then it is off to Frankfurt, Germany. Everything about this situation is out of my comfort zone because, first, I have a terrifying medical issue I have to combat and I'm leaving the comfort of my home to do just that. Second, I enjoy a regular and predictable routine. I have to admit I'm scared to be going to a foreign country for medical treatment, of all things, when for my whole career, I've worked for a major medical facility here in Florida. On the other hand, given my personal experiences with what I've seen for cancer treatments that didn't work at all and caused so much anguish, I feel I don't have a choice in this matter but to seek treatment elsewhere. I must trust God on this journey as His word says He is with me ALWAYS! I must also trust the medical staff I'm heading to that God will lead them as I have prayed, as well as the amazing research we have uncovered, thanks to my sister-in-law, Mary. We should arrive Saturday morning at 10am (that's 4am Florida time). Wish us well and keep us in your prayers.

Saturday, February 14, 2009 8:15 PM

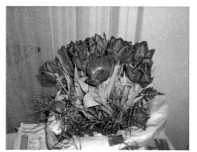

Happy Valentine's Day, German Style!

We are HERE! When we got to the room I found that Chuck had surprised me with a beautiful bouquet of Dutch red tulips and a Valentine's card in German! The plane flights were very uneventful and pretty enjoyable. It is very quaint up here with a little snow on the ground. The sun shined all day and the temp stayed in the 30's. We spent most of the day getting to the clinic and settling in. I had one local hyperthermia treatment along with 2 IV (intravenous) infusions, one high-dose vitamin C and one mixture of 3 different B vitamins.

Let me shortly explain the local hyperthermia treatment. The area where cancer cells were found, in the right axilla, is heated up to about 111 degrees F each day while I'm here. This is carried out by a machine that has an arm. (See picture of me getting this treatment on the page dated Feb. 17) At the end of the arm is a water-filled half-ball attached to the arm which is lowered to touch the skin. The water keeps the skin from burning while infrared rays are directed through the water and go deep into the tissues to heat the tissues underneath up to 8 inches deep. This heat damages the cancer cells while not harming healthy cells, which can handle the heat just fine. In my right breast there was a tiny 4 mm spot found, which they figured was the primary cancer site, so my local hyperthermia treatments will be alternated every other day to "hit" both the right breast and the right axilla . Sundays are a day of rest with no treatments.

We are pretty tired from our travels and are going to go to bed early. Remember, we are 6 hours ahead of Florida time. Sundays are a day of rest with no treatments. So tomorrow, only a couple of infusions, then we will be exploring the nearby town of Nidda.

Sunday, February 15, 2009 10:30 PM

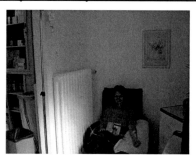

Prayers for Our Pastor from Abroad – Heart Attack

Thank you all so much for the words of encouragement you've given from home! It makes me feel like I'm not so far away.

We are completely rattled to hear that the Pastor of our church has had a heart attack and is in the hospital. He and the whole church have been so supportive of us. It's hard being so far away when things like this happen at home. We have been praying for him and will keep doing so. (Follow-up about Pastor Tom at the end of this book)

Otherwise, today was quite relaxing. We slept in and barely made it to breakfast as they were cleaning up. The food is healthy but not everyone "juices" like I do so I have asked Annette and Andrea in the kitchen for more veggies. Andrea walked me to the fridge in the back and told me to pick whatever I wanted. They are so kind and helpful here. Next, I had my 2 IV infusions of vitamin C and Bs. They use butterfly needles...tiny...Yay! Then we went walking to Nidda for about an hour. It's a cozy quaint little town. The temp is just below freezing so the snow is not melting at all. We have some great warm clothes and hats, thanks to all those who loaned us things!

We are meeting lots of wonderful people from all over the world. Here is where they are from; South Africa, Malta, Antigua, Germany of course, and the US (Colorado, Utah, Atlanta, Alabama, several cities in Florida, and Texas). Most everyone has tried conventional treatments at home, and then has found this place after their doctors told them there was nothing else that could be done for them. The patients say they wished they had come here first like I did. Tomorrow I will be busy, starting with lab work at 8 am, then an ultrasound, and then we'll be meeting with Dr. Herzog to discuss and make a schedule of my treatment plan for the next 3 weeks. OK, where is my massage and foot reflexology?

Guten Nicht! (Good Night!)

Monday, February 16, 2009 2:17 PM, CST

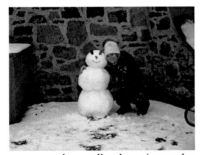

I'm a Krankenschwelter!

Monday is a lot busier than the weekend, as expected. When the nurse came in at 8 am to check on me she announced "it's snowing!" Being from Florida, we jumped out of bed and ran to the window. As you can see in the picture we enjoyed it a lot even before my treatments for the day started. It seemed we were the only ones enjoying the snow, and actually choosing to be out there!

Today I had bloodletting with leeches (a nice nurse drew blood with a tiny needle), an EKG (a simple heart screening), lung function test (130%, why am I here?), foot reflexology (squeeze those toesies massage), and a local hyperthermia to the right breast which was very hot this time! Felt like I got my money's worth, almost too much. The nurse said the local hyperthermia should be comfortable and "fussed" at me for letting it get to where it was hurting. If it burns my skin, she said, they can't do more hyperthermia there for a few days. Later, I found this to be a common occurrence with many other patients here, "grin and bear" the burnings to kill more cancer cells. But that's NOT how it works! Now I know.

At breakfast, when the cook brought to me a huge platter of raw veggies for juicing, everybody was staring and "oohing", and I heard someone say, "you're going to turn into a rabbit". Then a lady from Texas ran to me and asked how she could get that. Just ask, I said, but I shared my platter with her because they DID give me a lot!

Dr. Herzog came to our room, looked over all my supplements I brought from home and gave suggestions. He is very nice and soft spoken and said after the tests come back, he'll see me again. By the way, I learned today that I am a krankenschwelter, (the "w" is pronounced as a "v") the German word for "nurse"!

Tuesday, February 17, 2009 9:00 PM

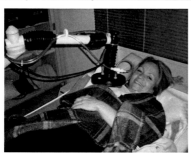

Thymus Injections

Guten Tag ("gooten tock") Good Evening!

This morning, bright and early, I was awakened with a "good morning" to a tiny, but quite burning injection to the tummy area. They have started Thymoject injections which will now be given by IV, thank goodness because it stung for an hour. Thymoject is a major immune booster which works by increasing the T-cells in the body which fight bacteria, viruses, and cancerous cells. Yes, I'll take more please!

I have been practicing some words in German and the nurses seem to like that I'm trying. They can actually understand me! I seem to be adjusting to my surroundings better, even though I am still way out of my "comfort zone". It's a 35 bed klinik so we now know practically everyone here and are just trying to remember names. We always have interesting conversations with other patients and their families and today was no different. At breakfast the two women we were talking with stated they have peripheral neuropathy (numbness, pain, and tingling) in their feet and legs from Taxol, a chemo given by their doctors "back home" in the US. They both require daily and/or weekly treatments to manage it but it's not going away. Both said their doctors either didn't tell them about that side effect or downplayed it when it occurred. This angers me. That's what my oncologist wanted to put me on at home. And he never said anything about that side effect either, just that Taxol was the easiest drug of the 3 I would be receiving! Treatments should not cause other health problems! The people here give me inspiration and some are so very sick from previous treatments. Yet still, their attitudes are that of gratitude and love for life. Most of the women here are being treated for breast and/or ovarian cancer....and most are from the US.

After breakfast, I had an ultrasound of my liver, right chest and axilla (will get results tomorrow) and received my vitamin C infusion, still getting stuck each day for that but it barely hurts; still using that baby needle! By then, it was time for lunch, which is the biggest meal of the day. I always start my meal with yucky juice, I mean, "healing juice". They ran out of carrots...I wonder why?

When researching German clinics we came across a blog of a couple who received treatment at this clinic. Well, we met them today! We read about their stay here, on the internet, even before we made plans to come, which made me feel more comfortable about traveling so far away for treatments in a foreign country. I felt like they were already my friends. They are a wonderful couple, but we were both busy with therapies so couldn't talk that much today.

We love going outside so we walked to the end of the town and checked on our snowman. He had fallen over on his face. I saved his arms for when we rebuild him. There's not much snow left but we should be getting more this weekend. Ok, my daughter will appreciate this random moment...I really miss everyone at home! Sniff, sniff. Ok I'm back.

There is a fully loaded gym here so I did some yoga and mini-trampoline jumping (moves around the lymph fluid thereby increasing the immune system). Then I had the dreaded... massage... poor me! After that was tea time at 3 where we did more visiting and met new people from Birmingham, AL and Nashville, TN.

It was then time for my Magnetic Field Therapy followed by an Ozone Intramuscular Injection (was dreading that all day). Between my knowledge of giving painless injections and the krankenswelter's (nurse's) expertise, I hardly felt a thing... wow! Very strange treatments. We included pics of various treatments throughout this book (not the ozone shot, it doesn't go into the arm!). This evening I had my local hyperthermia again to the right axilla (see picture) and fell fast asleep which is easy to do as the room was quiet and darkened and I had my cozy "blankie" from home. It lasted one hour.

Dinner was light as usual and now here I am on the computer again. I love having the computer here and reading the letters and notes from friends and family at home. Tonight, which is now at 9:30pm, we plan on using "skype" to see and talk with the family at home...yay! Again, thank you for the words of encouragement from home. They keep me going and I look forward to them every day!

Bis morgen (till tomorrow)

Wednesday, February 18, 2009 12:30 PM

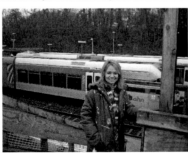

Three Little Angels

Today, I just started off tired, and then one of the doctor's couldn't start my IV for the infusion. As I was sitting there waiting for them to come try again there was an airplane out the window flying far off in the distance, I started feeling very homesick and missing everyone. I tried to hide that I was starting to cry.

When Dr. Herzog came in to talk about my treatment, I had a feeling he would mention low-dose chemo, which he did. Then I started to cry again. Well, he said when he gets the rest of the tests back tomorrow he will talk with us some more. 10 minutes later the massage therapist called our room and said they had an empty table waiting for me and can I come right now. Of course, I went right now. Dr. Herzog must have called them because I was not on the schedule for a massage today. That's one......

Chuck and I went to lunch, and missed it. Lunch was over... Chuck's watch was 45 min slow for some reason. We had an apple and nuts in our room instead.

We realized we needed some fresh air and wanted to take the train to Nidda. We ran into one of the patient's relatives from Alabama who was heading there to the post office. He was like a little angel for us and showed us where the train was, how to buy a ticket, when the train was returning, and just in case, how to walk back if we needed. He sat with us and showed us where to get off. We would have stayed riding since the ride there was so short. Once we were in the town, he showed us where the shops were and we split up. That's two......

We had an absolutely great time there with the beauty and quaintness of the cobblestone streets, the cute little shops, and the gorgeous sunny, cool weather. See the pic of Chuck and me having a beer and a hibiscus tea, respectively, in Nidda at the back of this book on the "About the Author" page.

We came back to the train station and missed it by 15 seconds! It stays on time always! Ok, we'll walk. The walk was fabulous...up and up and up a very steep, long, quiet road, then down the mountain. We went thru beautiful woods and fields right back onto street. Very exhilarating workout with such fresh crisp air!

Now, you would think I would feel better...well I'm trying. This is when I realized I needed to read some promises that God is with me always and I should not fear or worry. Now I just wished I had remembered that this morning. We need continued prayers for guidance, healing and encouragement, please. Some days I just feel like I'm teetering on the edge of "full out" crying.

This evening went much better with dinner, local hyperthermia, oxygen therapy, and then a successful needle stick with an infusion of lymphdiaral. We couldn't find much info in English about lymphdiaral. It must be a German thang! They said it gets the lymph moving around to increase the immune system and detox the body. There sure is a lot of that kind of therapy going on here!

After dinner one of the nurses came and whispered that she had left a note for me in my room. When we got back here, I found her note stating she had left a warm heating pack under the blanket for me (I have been requesting and using one for the last two nights for one of my treatments from home). What a sweetheart! Her name is Antje, short for "angel" I suppose. That makes three......

On an especially difficult day, "three angels" were sent to me to let me know that I am loved and cared for and through missing the train, we had a much needed opportunity to enjoy the beauty and splendor of the German countryside on a gorgeous day! God just likes to tap us on the shoulder sometimes and say, "Hey, I'm still here!"

So do not fear, for I am with you; do not be dismayed, for I am your God. I will strengthen you and help you; I will uphold you with my righteous right hand. Isaiah 41:10

Thursday, February 19, 2009 6:40 PM

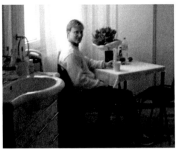

Needle in My Neck

Today wasn't quite as hard but I am very anxious about tomorrow. I know I shouldn't be after all my blessings from yesterday. As of yet, at 9 pm, I'm still waiting for Dr. Herzog to come and talk to us more about tomorrow. I will be having my first Whole Body Hyperthermia (WBH). It is fear of the unknown and as a nurse, not being in charge of the situation, that has me so uneasy. I have been getting lots of support from others who have gone thru it here. I actually forgot to go to my magnetic therapy and ozone injection today. Funny though, I didn't forget my foot massage...hmmmm.

Another reason I'm not thinking clearly today is because I had to get the IV placed in my neck jugular vein in preparation for tomorrow. That was nerve wrecking. Chuck held my hand and prayed the whole time (not out loud). I was praying too! Here's how they did it. You lay on an angle with your head low so the jugular vein in your neck pops up, then they numb the spot with a small needle. Then with ultrasound guidance they insert a needle into the vein which is then removed, but a flexible catheter is left in, taped securely, and bandaged. Now I have no more needle sticks for my daily infusions. What a relief! The procedure did not even hurt, surprisingly, but it's a little sore now and they gave me an ice pack and a mild pain reliever that I have not heard of...oh well, down the hatch. Sometimes you just have to be trusting..... After the huge calm I feel from getting through a scary procedure, I'm just not in the mood to figure out a pain pill! But they said that the procedure went perfectly and that I had "great jugulars"! Hadn't heard that one before!

Just to give an idea of what goes on in our room, Chuck is behind me watching a big German beer party on TV, what else would be on German TV? Very loud Germans, lots of colorful clothing and very loooong tables. I'd rather be there even with no beer. They are having so much fun!!! I love hearing them yell, "eins, twei, drei" (1,2,3) then they drink beer from huge, maybe half-gallon size, thick glass mugs. Those women carrying those full mugs to the tables have super strong "Hulk" arms! I am fascinated with their language and am learning some words. I feel like I am picking up their accent even with my American words! It's a very fun accent. In the 3 weeks I'm here I better learn something.

We haven't been outside today at all. I don't like that. It's gorgeous today, just cold. We've been hanging around for the doctor. We did go to the gym for more mini-trampolining and yoga and we opened the window in the room a lot. I suppose it's ok we're stuck in here, I needed to do some inspirational reading. They did add oxygen therapy which is breathing 3 liters/minute of pure oxygen for the hour that I'm getting my local hyperthermia treatment. Cancer doesn't like oxygen.

We have breaking news at the moment........

Dr. Herzog just left and he spent about **an hour and a half** with us, answering all our questions and giving us our options. There was no feeling to rush to a decision. He knew I was apprehensive about getting chemo. This shows what a wonderful, caring doctor he is. Who does that back in the states, and late at night?! Long story short for now, I will be getting a Valium to get a good night's sleep and my WBH hyperthermia tomorrow will be at 11 am here, or 5 am Florida time. I will be getting heated up to anywhere from 104 to 107 degrees F and we've agreed on low-dose chemo during hyperthermia session. I ask for prayers of protection from any short- or long-term side effects and for total healing. Through prayer, I am confident that God has lead us to this decision and Dr. Herzog is very confident in his treatment. I want to praise Jesus for my strength through all this and the Holy Spirit for constant guidance.

Friday, February 20, 2009 10:30 PM

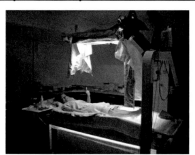

My First Whole Body Hyperthermia Treatment EVER!

I had quite the awaking this morning. This seems to happen a lot here! Never a dull moment! The nurse came at 7:15 am to prep me for my whole body hyperthermia. First it was the usual routine of blood pressure and oxygen level, next a finger prick to test sugar level. Then came the usual "clean out" typical of certain medical procedures. Finally, the starting of IV fluids. This is where that great jugular line in my neck comes in handy. Being such a large vein, it allows IV fluids to run into my body extremely fast and without any hesitation, unlike any veins in the arms. These fluids, which will have a little salt and sugar in them that are present in sweat, are necessary to keep my body hydrated, replacing copious amounts of fluids lost from sweating that goes along with a super high "fever". At 10:30 am we got the call to come down to the hyperthermia room to get started.

As stated before, through careful, prayerful consideration, I have decided to have Low-Dose Chemotherapy (LDC) with the whole body hyperthermia (WBH). I have always been against chemo because of the long-term effects they can cause, as well as the issue of healthy cells coming under siege and being destroyed along with the cancer cells.

The LDC course I will receive is made up of totally different drugs than those discussed back home. They are actually three older drugs. Dr. Herzog said his course is about 1/3 the strength of what is used in the U.S. and should have no short-term or long-term side effects, not even hair loss. The reason he can use such low doses is because of the hyperthermia. The heat, besides killing cancer cells, causes cancer cells to absorb much more chemo then they normally would as they are trying to survive. The heat also weakens the cancer cells making them more susceptible to destruction by the chemo. Hyperthermia increases the effectiveness of chemo by three times.

Another point the doctor made for adding the LDC was that due to the location, under the arm, of the affected lymph nodes, heat alone may not eradicate all of the cells. There are a lot of blood vessels located there and cancer cells may be able to hide and stay cool enough to survive even under the harsh hot conditions. The LDC treatment is used to finish them off, and any others in the body. I use the word "course" because I will be taking the LDC several times. Next Friday, eight days after WBH, I will have another round of LDC during my local hyperthermia treatment. This will provide a "kick 'em while their down" effect on the cancer cells, for total annihilation! I'm having this second treatment with local hyperthermia instead of WBH because a person can only go through one super heating (WBH) session about every one and a half to two weeks to allow for recovery from the stress of the heat as well as time for the body to rid itself of dead cancer cells, which is the reason to detox afterwards.

Thumbs up, I'm ready! (see picture)

I'm back!!! According to my husband, Chuck, here's how it all went down. The procedure lasted around four hours. I got a IV sedative which made me sleep through the whole thing. It generally takes about an hour and a half to slowly raise the body temperature to the desired goal. With me, their goal was to reach 105 degrees F, or more, and hold it there for at least an hour. Anything over 104.2 degrees F is considered "extreme" heat therapy. They were able to heat the core temperature of my body to 105.7 degrees F and hold it there for over an hour. Then, the heaters were turned off to allow my body to cool down naturally, and the sedatives stopped so I would wake up. It was such a soothing sleep that they had to wake me up and help me into the wheelchair. It generally takes a couple of hours for the body temperature to come back down to normal. I came through it with flying colors, so I'm told!

Afterwards, being wheel-chaired through the hallways of the clinic on the way to the recovery room, we wheeled by Chuck along with several of our new friends! Yikes, I can't imagine how I must look after being "drugged" and sweating for four hours! They didn't care! They were all full of cheers and smiling faces. What a great sight to see. They made my day! It was so nice to have that kind of support and camaraderie that comes from actually living at the clinic all together. Of course, we each have our own "hotel" room! At this point, upon awakening from the sedatives, I actually felt great, just very groggy from the whole ordeal. The nurse told me I did "wunderbar" (wonderful) and that they infused over three liters of IV fluids during the whole thing, which is normal. That's over ¾ of a gallon of liquid infused in 4 hours! It's necessary because of all the sweating. In recovery, I received another liter of fluids while I slept for a couple of hours. What a wonderful sleep I had in the recovery room. At that point, you don't want to eat or move or get up, or be bothered by anyone! After a few hours, however, my nurse had a different idea and said now it's time to eat and wouldn't take no for an answer. So she helped me sit up and I was served dinner in bed. I remember it was chicken and it was good, but I wasn't that hungry. They must have called Chuck to come get me because he showed up and walked me back to our room, only to have me fall asleep again. What a nice, warm, relaxing day it's been!

Tomorrow I will be starting a detox program to flush out the chemo and dead cancer cells from my body. Once I have been fully detoxed, I will spend the rest of the week focusing on building up my immune system again in order to prepare for the next LDC/local hyperthermia round next week. This protocol of detoxing was not offered or even discussed at home. Neither of us has ever heard an oncologist having a detoxing program followed up with an immune building program right after administering chemo. What a shame…..

Saturday, February 21, 2009 10:30 PM

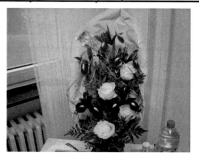

Thank you , Thank you, Thank you!

First of all, I need to address a few people. Aunt Frances, thank you soooo much for taking such good care of my family. You are an angel from heaven! Clarissa, I keep thinking about the encouraging words you've given me. And yeah, "hot mama" just about says it all after yesterday. Tanya, thank you for the wonderful "going to Germany" gift box. Kim B. thank you for the goodies for the trip. It all came in handy for the long travel day. Pastor Tom, a week after a heart attack and you're back to your usual silliness, thank God, literally! You keep on with those stupid letters. Just pretend no one else can read them. It feels so good to laugh and giggle as the stress of the day just melts away with a good belly laugh. Laughter truly is the best medicine!

Each night, both Chuck and I look forward to the amusing anecdotes and encouraging words from everyone at home. Sure helps us feel like we aren't so far away. The internet is a lifesaver for keeping us feeling close and in touch! Julie, thank you for checking on my family at home, and lending your daughter to play, and burp (if that's what you call that horrible noise), with my children! Mary, thank you for the uplifting support and admiration. Carey's mom, thank you for the long coat I've been wearing every day. Nancy, thank you for the warm boots. Pat, thank you for the warm furry hat and knit socks. Janice, thank you for the warm fuzzy ski stuff. Congratulations, Aunt Donnelleigh, I wish I could be home to see you and your new nephew. Rhonda, thank you for the dinners for my family at home...twice!!! Carmen, I wish I could be there to see your cute little dog, Max, with his pitiful little cast! All my neighbors thank you for taking care of my family while we are gone. My Aunt Frances is sooo appreciative of all of you and says how wonderful you all are!!! Doug, it's comforting that there's a guy here who talks and sounds exactly like you. It feels like you're here when I hear him. He lives in Texas but I'm not sure where he is originally from. Everyone, thank you for the wonderful words of support, silliness, and encouragement. I need it even more now I'm very homesick as the newness has worn off.

I came through yesterday just great. I don't remember much, except that it was all good. The day provided "blurry warmth" whose only rival is a day at the beach in Florida! Yes, it was that relaxing! The only proof I went through it is a little burn blister on my 2nd right toe and some puffiness all over. I felt wobbly earlier today but am feeling more normal now... just a little tired. There are a few people here that are going home tomorrow and I wish I was one of them.

Today went very smoothly with my magnetic field therapy, ozone shot, local hyperthermia, 2 infusions for immune boosting (Thymus and High dose Vit. C) and one for detoxing (the lymph solution). Those are a breeze now with this line in my jugular, which feels a lot better today. We had a fun dinner tonight. One of the nurses told a patient how to say something "nice" in German, then when she, the patient, said it to a cafeteria lady; we realized it wasn't nice after all. Just then, the nurse walked by and realized what had happened and got embarrassed. She said with a red face "it was just a joke"! What she was supposed to have taught her to say was "how may I help you" when really she taught her "what's your problem". Now, that turned our loud table into a super loud table as the roar of laughter continued. What fun! It sure is a roller coaster of emotions here and I love these "up" times.

I am trying to stay positive, which can be hard for me at times. There are sick people here and I don't want to be one.

Chuck got me more flowers today. They are yellow roses, gerbera daisies and tulips... beautiful. It really brightens up the room having flowers here. The red tulips were dropping petals like rain. Most of the patients here seem so upbeat. I don't know how they do it! They inspire me to try harder! I am meeting wonderful people here who are even uplifting me. I am starting to see them as warm loving people instead of "cancer patients" (I hate that term).

Here is something that one of my new friends, Becky, from Texas slipped under my door the night before my Whole Body Hyperthermia, about which I was very anxious. *"He giveth power to the faint, and to them that have no might he increaseth strength." Isaiah 40:29.* And this, her favorite verse as well as her email address since starting this journey herself, *"Now unto Him that is able to do exceeding abundantly above all that we ask or think, according to the power that worketh in us." Ephesians 3:20* She is a sweetheart and as hilarious as Lucille Ball in "I Love Lucy"! What makes her so funny is she doesn't realize she's so funny. She has us all in stitches many times a day!

Sunday, February 22, 2009 8:00 PM

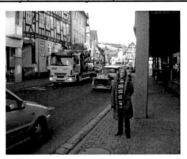

Carnival in Nidda

We just got back from downtown Nidda with Becky and Rodney from Texas. We didn't miss the train back this time. Good thing because it has been very cold... a wet and cloudy 42 degrees F and dropping. They had Carnival today. We missed the parade but saw all the confetti and trash and some pretty wild costumes. I took pictures of course while I sat having some chamomile tea at the cafe. After being at Mardi Gras, nothing shocked me, but Becky from Texas was... well, shocked by the wild costumes and masks and other paraphernalia worn by the locals. It was a welcome sight for me, being born in New Orleans, and having been to Mardi Gras there many times. It was also nice to get out and breathe fresh cold air after being inside for two days. I only had 2 infusions today. On Sundays everyone gets a break and there are no treatments. I don't have my usual appetite today for some reason. It could be the mild effects of the chemo, different tasting foods than what I'm used to, or just that I'm homesick. The food here at the clinic is decent but it's just not what I'm used to. I think I'll just juice tonight to give my stomach a rest... if that's what you call a rest!

Chuck got some German ice cream today in Nidda, walnut and chocolate. I tasted it... yum! I didn't get my own because I know I need an optimal diet to help me heal. Then some guy on the street tried to give me his extra beer he was holding. I guess he felt sorry for me that I didn't have either an ice cream or a beer! Amazing how God always sends something to laugh at or someone to make me laugh just when I need it! Lots of fun and laughter, it helps a person get through these tough times…….

We will be attending a small concert in the lounge here at the clinic tonight and plan on having more fun after that, as usual. Seems like a party every night here. I've been reading my books I brought whenever I'm having a difficult emotional time and checking my computer for notes from home.

Thank you Mary for the "Breakthrough" book by Suzanne Somers. It's wonderful and very informative on all aspects of natural health. I also have a book written by my friend, Donna Watkins, "Bought Free: A Story of Redemption", which I have already read once. I miss her so much already as she just recently moved to Chicago. And Leslie, thank you for the book "A Taste of Believing God" by Beth Moore. It's very inspiring and I finished it quickly but will read it again. There are times I feel so homesick, even though I'm actually having a good time here.

I'm still feeling a little tired today. It could be the cold, cloudy, wet, outside. That kind of day always makes me feel that way. I made myself do 10 minutes on the mini-trampoline and some ab crunches on the ball while holding supportive pressure on my neck (the needle area). The IV site is still a little sore but quite a blessing to have an easy way to get all those good immune-boosting and detoxing infusions… painlessly!

All of this is so life changing, I believe for the better. I've always been a person who appreciates the little things in life because that was instilled in me by my mom. But now, that appreciation is compounded many times over.

The time's come to mosey on down to see if there's something simple I can eat for dinner and what new and exciting ways I can juice. Can't wait!

Wir Lieben Sie! (We Love You)

Monday, February 23, 2009 11:30 PM

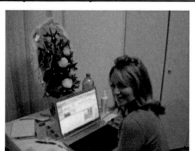

"Refiner's Fire" Poem & Juicing 101

We've been here over a week now and did I mention how much I miss home? I know a lot of people would love being away like this, but even as a child I've always been a "homebody", as in, I just love being at home. I even miss my heating pad. They do have really nice heating pads here but they have a peculiar smell, like a very strong essential oil, that I'm not crazy about. I would say I'm experiencing a slight aversion to strong smells like when I was pregnant, which I am not.

I use the heating pad for one of my own detoxing methods I learned from my holistic practitioner at home. A warm castor oil pack placed over the liver area of the tummy is a great detox for the liver. This organ is one of the largest detox organs of the body.

Another thing I found out is that the toxic aspect of my liver is one of the many reasons I got cancer in the first place. Looking back, I've really abused my health, mentally and physically, over the years. My poor self, "I'm so sorry and I will behave much better from here on out!"

I didn't eat most of the day today. Same situation as during pregnancy with taste changes and aromas. Eating strictly here at the clinic is kind of like eating at the same restaurant over and over again. I'm just getting tired of it. But Chuck is ok with it which tells me, it's me. We can't eat out because I need very healthy food, which is what they serve here. So today, I asked the chef for kidney beans for dinner tonight and they made a special bowl... just for me. It was like manna from heaven!! I must tell the chef how wonderful it tasted, he likes compliments!

Advice about juicing for those who want to incorporate more nutrition into their diets but don't know where to start, or can't get their family on board with them. I'm still working on trying to enjoy the "rich, full" flavors. I haven't really gotten to that point yet. It's all "ok" and tolerable, but the difficult part is the intensity of the flavors. For example, fresh carrot juice has about 10 times the flavor intensity as eating a raw carrot. That doesn't sound so bad until you start adding some "not sweet" vegetables. A good way of easing into juicing is to start light, such as juicing only apples, and even adding water to lighten it up. When that's comfortable, next time add one carrot, nothing else except maybe some water. Each time it goes well, add more carrots until the carrots and apples are in equal quantities. That's a great start. Other vegetables can be added a little at a time, over time. Berries are also very good and are low in sugar! But please, only organic for anything juiced.

For my personal juice recipe and how I used it when I first got "the diagnosis", as well as an explanation of the castor oil pack instructions and it's benefits, please visit my website at www.AHealthyApproach.com.

Today, I just shut down and slept most of the day. I guess I needed it because I'm feeling much better this evening. The nice massage therapist came to my room looking for me because I was sleeping and forgot my appointment. They are very caring here! I keep telling myself that even though I'm so homesick, this is so much better than it could be if I had stayed at home, in my comfort zone, for my treatment!!!

Tomorrow the clinic is organizing a trip to Friedberg to watch the Carnival parade (Mardi Gras, German style). It should be fun and a nice change of scenery.

I'm still enjoying all the Valentine's cards I received from friends at church. I read them slowly, enjoying every word to "savor" them, not wanting them to end. Mary D., I read your letter last night and am so touched at you suggesting "Jean day" (everyone wearing jeans for the day) in my honor at your work. You work with some very wonderful people! And Faith, thank you for the angel pin. I read your letter after I had sent the following message to my friend here, Becky. Poor Chuck, every time he turns around, I'm crying for some reason or another. Homesick, grateful, relieved, happy.....whatever. They all call for tears!

I continue to read scriptures and my uplifting books. I could not do this without them and Chuck!! My friend had her Whole Body Hyperthermia today so I visited her in her room. We were talking and laughing and, being a nurse, observing her "pee" bag (sorry all you non-medical people out there) and checking out her IV's since I wasn't alert enough to check out my own on my "special" day. She had lots of questions about her IVs so I proceeded to explain to her about the ones I knew. They have totally different drugs here so Chuck and I look up everything. It's all so interesting! In fact, one of my own IVs was new so we looked it up. It was just another "detox"... speed 'er up, Charlie! Bring it on! Back to my friend, her BP (blood pressure) was very low after her WBH and she was nervous about that. Knowing I'm a nurse, she asked me if she was going to be ok. Another thing she does that's cute, she over-reacts and worries about everything! She was on dopamine, which I explained how it increases her BP, and told her about how her kidneys are still fine with a BP above 60 over 40, which was where she was. Also, that the urine in the bag looked great! The look on her face told me I shocked her. She's one of those proper southern girls! I told her that one of the meds they gave her during the WBH has most likely caused the low BP and as soon as it gets out of her system she will be fine. We laughed, compared favorite scriptures and had some tears of joy and some stories for each other. So as usual, my good friend made me laugh until my stomach hurt, even in her recovery.

I sent the poem below to her email so she would have it when she got back to her room from Hyperthermia. It's from my book, "Bought Free: A Story of Redemption" by Donna L. Watkins, please read it carefully, it means a lot to me (as well as being very appropriate for the treatments we are receiving here!)

The Refiner's Fire

Sometimes the way God calls us to walk
We think it just can't be,
He didn't mean this, for after all
It seems too hard for me.

But all of us go through the fire
A refiner's fire so hot.
So God can check the purity
Of this lump of gold He's got.

It would be so much easier
If He took us to the heights
Where there is always love and peace
And we live within His light.

But as we go through the fire
He's walking there with us,
Teaching us to depend on Him
And learning more to trust.

He never sends us there alone
Or without a purpose clear.
He wants our best to always show

As we shine for those so dear.

So, in this hard time, trust Him
For He will see you through.
He'll never leave or forsake you
And you will be tried and true.

And because He is your Father
Who knows what's best for you,
You can rest within His loving arms
To see what great thing He'll do.

So as you walk beside Him
In this dark and lonely place,
Remember always, just look up
And you'll see His loving face.

I sent her this verse as well... *"For I know the plans I have for you," declares the LORD, "plans to prosper you and not to harm you, plans to give you hope and a future." Jeremiah 29:11.*

Tuesday, February 24, 2009 9:00 PM

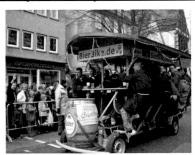

Friedberg Trip for Carnival!

This morning's note! I had my usual daily therapy including local hyperthermia, magnetic field therapy, ozone shot, and detox/immune boosting infusions. We'll be leaving shortly to go to Friedberg, about 15 kilometers (about 10 miles) from here, by van, from the klinik (clinic) for Carnival. I'm feeling a little weak, no appetite but the Dr. has prescribed a few "things" for me to help with that. He always has some great "tricks up his sleeve". One is to go to Carnival and yell "hal-ew". He says that will get my platelets up?

Speaking of my platelets, they were 62,000 yesterday and 73,000 this morning... going up! Supposed to be at least 150,000. Trying to figure out anything else that will make them go up. I'm splurging today and having a small, unsweetened cup of cafe au lait (a New Orleans coffee) and Dr. Herzog gave me an "apertif", which is a small medicinal "liquor" for my appetite. I've lost another kilogram in the last 3 days. Down to 120 lbs. That's a very healthy weight for me and I actually look fabulous. My color is great even without makeup! I've got my bright purple turtleneck on and Dagmar, the nice nurse, just came in and said the van will be leaving shortly. Gotta go, will let you know how the day went.......

Evening time and we are back from our outing. I'm so wiped out! It was quite cold out there and I had all the warm clothing on that I had brought. My stomach became a little upset on the van ride there. There were a lot of winding roads and they drive pretty fast here. Combining that with a slight chemo stomach just put me over the edge. I wanted to have fun so bad. I kept praying for relief. "Just 10 minutes" if nothing else. The day was beautiful, sunny and crisp.

The parade was a lot like the Mardi Gras parades in New Orleans except the floats were smaller (but the same amount of drinking going on….a lot) Notice the beer keg on the front of the float in the picture! And the crowd yells "hal-ew" instead of "throw me somethin' mister", and they throw Haribo Gummi bears and confetti from the floats instead of Moon Pies and beads, like in New Orleans.

After about an hour into the parade they started throwing, of all things, German saltine crackers! I started nibbling on one and... it helped my stomach! I don't believe in coincidence. Thank you, God! I was able to enjoy the day more. Later, we all had some drinks (no alcohol for me) in a "happenin' café" along the parade route... I just ate more crackers, and the ride back was just fine.

I think I'm coming down with something because I felt achy all over and fever-ish, jumping into bed as soon as we got back. The nurse gave me some liquid for my nausea, then I took a nice warm nap. She also offered me another "apertif" which I didn't need. I had ordered red beans and brown rice for dinner which was again, fabulous, and very appropriate for Mardi Gras!

After eating my marvelous, Mardi Gras dinner, I felt much better and we started watching a movie on Chuck's computer in our room... "Relative Values". It's supposed to be funny. My sweet nurse, Antje, will be bringing me some vapor rub and hot water for an inhalation therapy before bed since I feel a cold coming on. She takes good care of me.

Wednesday, February 25, 2009 11:00 PM

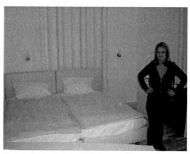

Washing Clothes, German Style

Today was yet another day of rest. This place sure does well for lowering the stress of everyday life. A quaint little town away from the "rat race" of home with not much to do except concentrate on getting well. There's only that internally produced stress of doubt that keeps hanging around.

I had my local hyperthermia treatment, three IV's, another detoxing procedure, and message therapy. My platelets are up to 82,000, and rising, but still not high enough to have my low-dose chemo this Friday. Instead, Dr. Herzog has ordered that we use the weekend to get out and explore some of the local German hospitality.

Chuck washed clothes today while I was resting. Again, this place sure does well for lowering stress! One has to be very careful with the washer and dryer. Instructions are all in German. With the washer, if you're not careful with the settings, your clothes can wash as long as 360 minutes (6 hours)! The dryer does not have a vent. There is a tray that collects water as it evaporates from the clothes. If it's full and you forget to empty it before you start the dryer, your clothes will never dry. "Wery Intervesting, but not vunny" (an old "Laugh-In" joke for those old enough to remember).

As I said earlier, Chuck did the laundry and I rested most of the day. Unfortunately, I've been fighting a pretty bad sinus cold that's made me feel like I have the flu, like I'm dying! Fever, achiness, and extreme weakness. Even though it was a very nice, sunny day today, we decided I needed a lot of rest and sleep so I could kick this cold fast. To help fight it, Dr. Herzog prescribed inhalation therapy using chamomile tea. In a basin of very hot water, chamomile tea bags are added, then you lean over it, with a towel covering your head, and inhale the vapors. A very weak tea, not quite boiling, is best since it did cause me to cough when I stayed there too long breathing in very deeply. I tend to overdo something if I think it's going to help. Hot boiling water and very strong tea, inhaling very deeply until it burns! Don't do that. He also gave me an intravenous "Cold Cocktail" containing three homeopathic and Sinupret Forte tablets.

Sinupret Forte is a sinus medicine, developed in Germany that is made of four herbs. Most of the herbs in it, I have heard of, and are known for boosting the immune system. It has worked really well with my coughing and sinus pain. Being herbs, I'm not having any side effects from it (sleepiness, sleeplessness, dry mouth, too dry of a nose, etc). I love it! I found out that it can be purchased online and is available at Walgreen's at home! I'm actually feeling a little better tonight and hope to be able to get out and about tomorrow. What a huge change from how I felt just this morning!

Tyler, it was really nice reading your message. I guess even Jack, our dog, is going through withdrawals with us being gone. He's never chased a mailman before! Again I wanted to thank everyone for your support and the encouraging messages. They really, really mean a lot to us. We love you all and miss everyone.

Pictured above is how we arranged our beds so we could sleep by each other. Otherwise, the twin beds were divided by a nightstand. It's all about support these days! The rooms are simple, very clean, and quite comfortable with large windows looking out on the countryside. Every room has a beautiful, healing view!

Thursday, February 26, 2009 10:00 PM

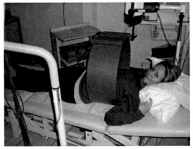 # Info on my Two Chemotherapy Drugs

Today has been a lot more cloudy then yesterday and I'm still fighting off the sinus cold which has wiped me out so much I can barely even think. I slept until around 10:30 am, waking only to have my three infusions started. There was no lab work ordered until tomorrow, so no report on my platelets. We ate lunch in our room because Dr. Herzog was due to visit us around 12:30 pm. For some reason, my feet have been cramping for the last couple of days so he prescribed some magnesium pills. Other than that, Dr. Herzog said everything looks good.

Now that it's evening time, I'm beginning to have a little more energy again. The turning point for that seemed to be right after my massage by "Max". Wish I could get one of those every day! My massage went longer than usual, because, it seems Max loves Carnival and was fascinated that I have been to Mardi Gras in New Orleans many times and was even born in New Orleans. He wants to go there someday. We had fun comparing German to traditional Carnival. When he went to carnival here, he said he went as a "cowboy" this year. I told him that this year in Germany, I went as a "Freezing American". That gave him quite a laugh! He speaks fluent English with a great Germany accent. He told me that it's a standard subject in schools here, therefore, most young people can speak English. That's very forward thinking!

For treatments today I had had magnetic field therapy (see picture), an ozone shot, and local hyperthermia treatment. When I got done with my treatments I headed back to bed for another 2 hour rest. We ate dinner in our room again and watched Around The World In Eighty Days on Chuck's laptop since the TV does not have a DVD player.

I'd like to give some info on the two chemotherapy drugs I'm receiving here. Vinorelbine and Mitomycin, are the two low-dose chemo drugs. Mitomycin is actually a chemo "antibiotic". It is mildly toxic when used in standard chemo therapy. However, when it's used in combination with heat (Whole Body Hyperthermia) the toxicity increases three-fold or more! It becomes a highly toxic chemo drug to cancer. Once the heat is removed, Mitomycin returns to a mildly toxic medication. This is why Mitomycin can be such an effective chemo drug, as effective as the very toxic ones I was to be given at home, but have very little short-term side effects and practically no long-term side effects. Vinorelbine is also one that increases in strength when heat is added, yet at the same time, isn't very toxic to the body as the heat is removed. Pretty smart, those Germans.

The next several days are focused on detoxing, getting the chemo drugs out of the body as well as helping the body to flush out all the dead cancer cells, now that the damage to the cancer cells has been accomplished. Immune-boosting is also an important aspect of treatment, in order to assist the body in healing itself. All of this is accomplished through various IV infusions. This helps to ensure as few as possible, short- and long-term, side effects. Maybe one day these treatments will be added to routine cancer treatments offered in America.

I hope to feel more energetic tomorrow and we may try to do some shopping in Friedberg after my morning therapies. Again, thanks to everyone at home for the emails of support and encouragement.

I need to mention how special and loved I feel each day as I read the 24 Valentine's Day cards my friend Donna gave me as we headed off to Germany. One, written for each day that we would be away from home! I'm so tempted to read them all at once. It must have taken hours to put together. I will cherish them forever and read them again each Valentine's Day to remind me of the importance of wonderful friends and God's work in my life. Each card, which is in her own handwriting, contains a scripture of promise and a personal, beautiful prayer from her own heart. Each one makes me know that I am so loved and cared for by my wonderful friends and my forgiving, loving, and merciful Lord.

Friday, February 27, 2009 1:00 AM

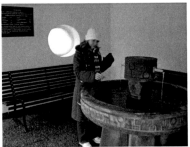

Mineral Springs

Sometimes we have so much fun here that it interferes with my sleep! But again, laughter is awesome medicine! Tonight we watched one of my favorite movies here with some friends. It's the 4th night in a row it's been watched by others, Chuck started it! I laughed for 2 hours. I need to watch it every day until I leave. The movie was "Rat Race". It seems to be funnier every time, and even more so when watched with friends. Between that and messages from friends at home, I'm laughing and feeling comforted daily!

Thank you so much for the laughs, the verses of promise, the reminders of healing, the updates from home, and just being there for me and my family. I'm so grateful for so much support. Chuck and I read them aloud each night so we both can laugh and be comforted….

This afternoon, I really started "perking up" as far as my energy level. The stomach thing, appetite, is still not quite there yet but getting better each day. My stomach actually growled today for the first time in days! That was exciting… it really was!

Chuck and I took a long walk in the mineral springs park, across the street, for about an hour. It felt great to get out again. We sampled from 4 different springs that all tasted differently depending on the elements contained in each one. They're all "fountained" up with a fancy spout and/or little house built around them and labeled with the elements contained in each. Dr. Herzog said the Lithiumqwelle (lithium well – see picture) was very healthy for white blood cells. We drank about a half cup of that one and just tasted the others. The flavor is so strong that one can't drink very much at a time. It tasted salty with a bit of a metallic taste but not too bad.

Another water well tasted very metallic and one was very salty and pungent tasting. Very unusual, I've never seen or heard of anything like these before. There is a huge inhalation area where salt is made and the vapors that come off of it are "medicinal". There are benches to sit all around it and breathe in the healthy vapors. Unfortunately, they can't run it during winter because the water would just freeze, as it trickles over huge "bundles of sticks" housed in an outdoor structure in the park.

My platelets are 126,000 today, praise God, and my white blood cells came down just a bit to 2.5, from 3.5. I'm due for one of the chemo drugs on Monday in combo with local hyperthermia. The doctor will give me a white cell booster if needed.

I wanted to share with you a story of a young Australian woman we met, who just left here yesterday in good health. She came to the klinik with cancer in her breast, lymph nodes, stomach, lung, and covering her liver. She was so ill and weak she almost didn't survive the plane trip on her first trip to the klinik. The doctors in Australia said there was nothing else they could do for her. Once she arrived here, even Dr. Herzog was extremely concerned about her condition. After two trips to the klinik, totaling about 11 weeks (this was her second trip), all of the cancer was gone except for 3 small spots on her liver. Dr. Herzog said that those areas should continue to shrink and turn into scarring. It was very encouraging for us to have actually met, not just hear about, someone who went from being extremely ill with a hopeless diagnosis, to being happy, full of energy, and with a bright future. I watched as she skipped down the hallway and bounced into the van that would take her to the airport to return home. Her husband was almost in tears as he excitedly explained that Dr. Herzog had saved her life.

Well, I must go to bed now if we are to get any sightseeing done tomorrow. And maybe some German pastry sampling!

Saturday, February 28, 2009 8:00 PM

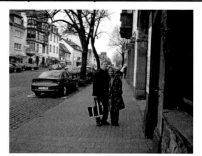

Shopping in Friedberg with Friends

I'm finally realizing that I feel much better if I just take the nausea drops Dr. Herzog gave me, a few times a day. Then I can have some fun and not cringe when it's meal time. I felt good enough today to head over to Friedberg, where Carnival was held on Tuesday, for some shopping. But first, I had 3 infusions and my local hyperthermia. Next, was lunch and I was treated to a surprise. Chuck had bought me a bouquet of white roses and purple lilacs, "just because". Beautiful! The picture of the bouquet is on the page dated Feb. 23, 2009.

After lunch, we got a driver from the clinic to take us, a friend, and one other couple to Friedberg so we wouldn't have to wait on the train or risk missing it. It's about 30 minutes away. He dropped us off right in the middle of the shopping district which was great (pictured). Otherwise, it would have been a long walk from the train station. We were in Friedberg for 2 and a half hours. We stopped in a little bakery and had these little poppy seed, soft pretzel balls. Delicious, but I only had one. They were the size of a large donut hole. What I was "eyeing" was the dark chocolate covered banana bread!!! Decadent, but I resisted! My health is more important right now.

Back at the klinik, during Dr. Herzog's daily visit, we asked him about Mistletoe Therapy (Iscador). We had read a lot about it being given in Germany to fight cancer. He said I would be receiving that at a later time. Right now I'm receiving Thymus (Thymoject) which I will be continuing at home for a time. It's a small dose about the size of an insulin injection. The needle is pretty painless but the Thymus does sting a little.

He first prescribes the Thymoject, which is an immune support/booster during the active phase of treatments. He said it's better to support, or boost the body's immune system while receiving treatments, instead of actively stimulating the immune system at this time. Then, once things are "taken care of", he prescribes Iscador, the immune stimulator. Iscador will supercharge my immune system to become strong on its own and better able to fight off any potential re-occurrence.

After another walk in the beautiful park across the street, we're realizing that the taste of the water from the Lithium well seems to be stronger each time. We'll see how many times we can keep that up.

Tonight will be another relaxing dinner followed by a movie, hopefully. Even though it can be stressful going through cancer treatment, it's nice to be able to relax and laugh while we're here. It's been a really great day.

Sunday, March 1, 2009 11:00 PM

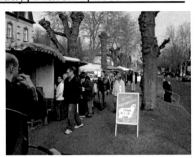

Farmer's Market in Town

We're on the home stretch now for this trip! We will be flying home next Sunday and will arrive at Orlando Int'l Airport at 10 pm...yay!!!!!!!!!! Today was a restful and fun day. I didn't get up until noon and then one of the doctors came in to check on me and see if I had any concerns or questions. I guess Dr. Herzog can have one day off. I had 2 infusions for detoxing and am taking the nausea drops even though my stomach feels good... just in case. Tomorrow afternoon during my local hyperthermia at 3:20 pm (9:20 am Florida time), I will be receiving one of the two low-dose "kimo" meds I received on Friday. "kimo" is how Kendall, my daughter's friend, wrote "chemo". I actually like that better, as I've never been a fan of chemo anyway, and don't like to write about it knowing it's referring to me. So, this is how I will be spelling it from now on. Thank you for lightening things up, Kendall!

I ask for special prayers at that time for "warrior strength" results. I may have a little uneasy stomach again after a few days. Hopefully my white blood cells will be ok in the morning. I'll just pray and then the right things will be done. I do have a massage at 9:30 in the morning which should get me off to the right start for the day anyway.

Back to the "restful and fun day" part. There's a Farmer's Market (see picture) on this street once a month and it was today. What luck that it's while we're here! It was similar to the one at home with food and flowers and gifts. We got some dried fruit, nuts and seeds for the trip home! As well a little German gift for Evan. It's a small 1 inch tall birdhouse that "chirps" when you twist it on its base. It does sound amazingly like a real bird. There are so many birds here in this little town that sing constantly all day long, that it seemed so appropriate. I also bought a scarf for myself.

Then we went to a cake shop across the street called "Haus Ira". It's only open on Sunday and Tuesday. I got a Hibiscus Tea and Chuck got a strong coffee. We split a piece of their special 4-layered almond cake that was covered with a light, delicious, "real whipped cream" frosting and filling... I allowed myself many, very small bites. Dr. Herzog said stuff like that every once in a while is fine. That it's good for the soul! I have to agree.

While we were sitting there, we heard sirens for the first time here so we hurried out and got pictures of the fire trucks whizzing by. We're such tourists! Their fire trucks are tiny and cute. Tiny Streets = Tiny Fire Trucks. Then we walked across the street to the park for my daily dose from the Lithium well. The whole time we were walking, there was a huge "glider plane" overhead just enjoying the day. I wanted to be up there so bad. It was close enough that we could hear the "whistling" sounds of the air going over the wings! Beautiful! We walked for over an hour. The weather was sunny with some clouds and around 44 degrees F, so we only needed a jacket and gloves. No face masks required today!

My nurse Antje (pronounced, Angie) just came in to say good evening. This is her last night before vacation so we got a picture and she showed us her family on the computer. She has a daughter, and is married to a Feuerwehrmin (Firefighter). What a sweetie.

Someone had a question from home asking what our son, Evan, was saying, when he wrote this to us. "At school I dekrated my kort. Love EVAN" Here's the translation, He "decorated" his milk "carton". They're making what's called a "Gingerbread Village" in 2nd grade, which is a town made out of milk cartons. They learn how a city works and how to spend money wisely on decorations and purchases. I'm so glad I'll be home to see the finished project in the classroom. It's a big thing for them that is weeks in the making.

Monday, March 2, 2009 10:45 PM

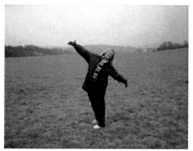

The Long Giggly Hour

Today was my foot massage first thing this morning... nice. My blister on my toe from the Whole Body Treatment is finally healed enough. We hung out in the room for Dr. Herzog's visit and he said my platelets are 172,000 now (so that's not an issue anymore) and my white blood cells are holding at 2.5 (normal is 4-10). He said he will check them again on Wednesday since I would have kimo today. We walked a lot in the park, drank Lithium water and I did a "Julie Andrews" on the hilltop (see picture). That was fun.

Then it was time for my low dose "kimo" treatment combined with local hyperthermia to my right axilla (underarm). Because I had to raise my right arm up for the local hyperthermia, my infusion kept stopping. We figured the line was kinked in my neck area, so Chuck had to hold the infusion line straight by pulling on the line over my chest for the whole hour. I had to keep my head turned to the left also, or that would make it stop too! This was all very awkward so I ended up laughing, which made the nurses laugh, which then caused Chuck to make even more jokes than usual. It sure helped with the stress of knowing kimo was being infused into my body.

To add to the distraction..... just 15 minutes into the hour-long session, I realized I needed to "pee" really bad! Of course, Chuck now tried to make me laugh even more. The whole hour was spent just trying not to giggle, which makes a person giggle all the more! I hope to be still giggling by Wednesday when the queasy feelings may start. All I can say is, I was praying for strength to get through this day. I didn't like "seeing" the kimo dripping into my body. The uncontrollable laughing was definitely a distraction. Leave it to God to turn a stressful situation into a humorous one.

Right after my treatment we went to the media room and watched a movie, which made me sit and relax so I got sleepy. It was cute and funny…"Out-of-Towners" with Goldie Hawn and Steve Martin. When I finally got back to my room and turned the computer on, I found that my nurse Antje just invited me to join her on my Facebook page, which I did, of course! I told her about our silliness during my local hyperthermia and kimo "combo". I'm sure she wishes she could've been there instead of off work, yeah right!

Early tomorrow morning, 7:40 am, I'll have a second local hyperthermia treatment to my right breast area while the "kimo" from today is still circulating in my body. Then in the afternoon, I'll start my IV detox regimen… definitely something to look forward to.

Tuesday, March 3, 2009 11:45 PM

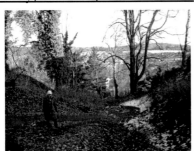

Beautiful Day in Nidda

Chuck and I had a very fine day today. All of my treatments were finished by 10:00 am. Dr. Herzog came to see us and we spoke about continued care and follow-ups. We will be getting more details at the end of the week.

Right after lunch we decided to go back to the nearby town, Nidda, and go to some of the shops since they were open today. Shops are not open for very long hours in Germany and most of them are closed between 12 and 2 for lunch. Then they close at 6 pm. Weekend hours are even less. People don't shop long hours here like they do in the U.S. Another thing we noticed is that there are no huge cars or SUVs on the roads. We were able to have the driver from the klink here, take us to Nidda since we missed the train by 2 minutes. I wasn't sure if I could walk the whole way, then make it around town, too, you know, with kimo yesterday and all. The day was gorgeous and sunny… around 50 degrees F… very pleasant compared to 18 degrees F. We stopped at a restaurant and just had drinks. My tea of choice today was "green"… The atmosphere was very quaint and comforting. We got a few gifts here and there and decided I felt so good that we would just walk back… up, up, up, the hill, then down and down back to our street (see picture). It was a good 30 minute hike… exhilarating, just like last time. I guess I still felt great, after all.

After we got back, we finally got to meet the wonderful lady, Vera, who helped us with getting our appointment here at the klinik. She visits here about once a month to meet those, in person, that she has assisted in getting here. We were one of those people. She comes from Munich and helps match people to the right klinik that she feels will suit their needs best. She is a wealth of knowledge and has a PhD in something, it can be hard to follow along with her accent. But anyway, she is fascinating to talk to. She's German and moved to the U.S. at age 19. She used to work in the cancer hospitals in California, and then New York, before moving back to Germany to start her business of helping spread the word about the German cancer kliniks. She did this because she didn't like what she saw with cancer treatments in the U.S.

We, and another couple, sat and talked with her for hours then took her out to dinner at a fancy hotel on our street. We all enjoyed a delicious restaurant meal and the atmosphere was quite luxurious.

With the early morning start I had today, I thought surely I would get in a nap today. Guess not! Places to go, people to see!

Wednesday, March 4, 2009 1:00 AM

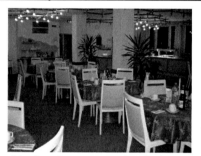

Nursing Lesson: Ask Questions!

My treatments were first thing this morning which consisted of 2 detox infusions (Lymphdiaral and L-Carnitine) and my local hyperthermia, and that was it. I then dragged myself outside, across the street with Chuck, to the Lithium well for some healing waters. Through it all, all I could think of was, "Why am I so very tired. I can't seem to shake off this sleepiness even after being outside in the nippy coolness of the day?" I decided not to fight it, caffeine is not an option, nor anything else which may hinder my healing. That's one of the many nice things about being here. There's that opportunity to just concentrate on your health without a thousand other obligations. So instead of sightseeing or shopping or walking, I decided to nap. However, upon awakening, I realized I'd slept for 5 hours! That was so much more needed than a few cups of coffee! I didn't even have lunch.

Dr. Herzog came in and woke me for the daily check. He did not have my lab work from this morning and I was too tired to ask for it. There will be plenty of time for that later. They are checking my white blood cells, red blood cells, and platelets. I told him that my feet were cramping again like last week and he put me back on magnesium. It really helped last time. As a side note, I'm looking forward to sleeping in my own bed soon. These beds are a bit hard for me, but comfortable. I'm a "super soft, squishy kind of bed" person.

Now, for that nursing lesson. Just like in hospitals in the U.S., you have to ask questions and get answers about your care, or have someone do it for you if you're not capable. Have the medical personnel write down words that you're not sure of the spelling, and understand what they are giving you and what it's for.

I'll share a couple of examples from my visit here, which are no different than any other hospitals I've ever been to, or worked in, over the years. The fact is, well over **70,000 people in U.S. hospitals alone** die each year due to medical errors, none of which I have ever caused, by the way! This is by no means meant to say they aren't competent here, because they very well are! This little lesson is meant to say, from nurse to patient, always be aware, and be involved with your care.

So, here are the examples, none of which would have killed me, by the way! The first day I was here, the nurse gave me someone else's pain med which I did not take because I didn't know what it was. When I asked about it she realized it wasn't for me. Another morning, the nurse was not aware I had lab work ordered and needed to draw my blood. Lab work is drawn before any infusions are given for the day. I insisted she draw my blood, which she did, because I knew I was due for lab work. And I was right. Tonight, I asked for my magnesium (Dr. Herzog said he was going to order it) because they hadn't brought it, which meant it would be included in tomorrow's meds. But I knew the feet cramps would waken me during the night if I didn't get it now, so I insisted until I got it. Don't get me wrong. They are very good nurses here, but nurses are still human.

In summary, don't be afraid to ask questions and be insistent until you're proven wrong, or until you feel satisfied with the answer. Ok, that's all for now. Everything has really been very good here as far as care and the nurses' desire and ability to help. Everyone knows, nurses (me) make the worst patients! But from what I've seen in the hospitals over the years, I feel that's the safest way to be.

After my all-day nap, we had dinner (see picture of cafeteria) with Vera de Winter again, the lady I spoke of last night. She is so fascinating and full of stories that we stayed talking with her until 10 pm tonight. And she loved the audience, us!

I received the medications from the pharmacy today, for taking home on Sunday. One is an "injectable", the Thymoject for immune boosting. I will need to give it to myself twice a week. I guess I can handle it. It's just a tiny needle. Do what ya gotta do, right?

Thursday, March 5, 2009 12:30 AM

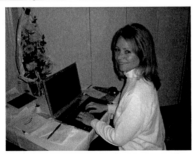

Game Night

Today was typical with local hyperthermia and infusions, foot reflexology (acupressure on the feet), which can be uncomfortable at times, but very therapeutic, also electromagnetic field therapy and ozone shot. My daughter says, "so that's where the ozone layer is going"! I also got a calcium infusion for my crampy feet and bone health, of course. We can't wait to come home. Did I already say that?

Dr. Herzog came in for his daily visit just before lunch. My white blood cells were up to 3.1 (they were 2.5 on Monday) and my platelets were up to 218,000 (172,000 on Monday). I noticed that he was still giving me Echinacea and is sending me home with liquid Echinacea. I asked him why I was still being prescribed it. He said that Echinacea helps to increase your body's white blood count. I always wondered exactly how Echinacea helped your body fight off colds.

We met another interesting couple today. They are from Iran, Medhi and Batoole. They speak perfect English. They are a very nice couple and we had a really good talk (even mentioned God in our conversation). Unfortunately, the way Iranians are portrayed by the media makes them all sound hateful and prejudiced. And here we are, having this huge "thing", cancer, in common.

Tonight we got to kick back and play a game called "Uno Spin" with some friends. Suddenly, in the middle of the game, it hit me and I said to everyone there, "Can you believe we're in Germany playing Uno Spin?" It was one of those moments where we all just sat back and pondered. What an odd adventure we're all having. The Uno Spin instructions were in German but our friends said they knew the rules so we had to believe them. Guess who won... hum....Surprisingly, they did!

I'm trying to make the days go faster but it's just not working! Sometimes it feels I'm walking in quicksand as far as how long these 3 weeks have been. My being a huge "homebody" makes it feel like we've been here for 6 months. Chuck, on the other hand, is doing just fine! I think he's enjoying being away from home. He's even able to do work from here on his computer. I'm sure he'd rather be working from Germany (exciting) than Florida (blah).

I love reading messages from home and hearing about things going on nearer to my part of the world. It gives me that connected feeling and helps with the home sickness. We saw the family again on SKYPE tonight (live video conferencing). With the time being 6 hours ahead, we can't stay up every night to see them. I REALLY dislike it when it's time to say "goodbye". I love seeing their little faces and hearing their sweet little voices and laughter. Sigh……..

Again, I am so grateful to everyone who has checked in on my family and made dinners for them as well as giving us words of encouragement and prayers! The help from my friends and family has been so amazing. The only repayment I could ever begin to make would be to pass along any help to others as often as I could, forever!

Friday, March 6, 2009 10:15 PM

Almost Home at Last!

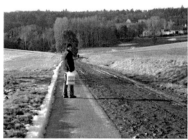

This trip here is winding down. I have been energetic and looking forward to early Sunday morning when we leave for the airport. I have an early morning appointment tomorrow at 7:30 am for my local hyperthermia and infusions, and also requested and extra magnetic field therapy and ozone injection. What was I thinking? I should have requested an extra back massage! I am still receiving detox and immune boosting infusions each day. I feel those are so important in the whole aspect of healing.

As already stated, we're getting some good exercise and rest here. We walked back from Nidda again (see picture)... up up up the hill and down down into town. Although it's not noticeable in the picture, it's quite a steep hill and very exhilarating. It really gets the blood moving and that fresh, unpolluted air fills the lungs! It was a cold sprinkling rain but we were well dressed and nicely warm. We could have taken the train but I wanted to walk. That walk is one of my favorites here. We took a luxurious nap before dinner.

I'd like to "recharge my batteries" before the flight home, which is tiring with the long hours and the 6 hour time zone difference. I think everyone should take afternoon naps, a requirement, like when we were in kindergarten.

I want to mention that I do have follow-up visits here. They won't be 3 weeks though. This is the toughest trip, only because of the length of time away from home. I would like, more than ever, for this whole ordeal to be over-with on Sunday when we leave. However, there are times when persistence is key, and this is one of them. I will need to return so that I can finish my "series" of low-dose kimo treatments, combined with one whole body hyperthermia and local hyperthermia's each day. Of course, I'll have all the infusions and detox therapies that go with it. The next visits will only be about 10-12 days. That, I can do more easily. Dr. Herzog spoke with us this week about returning so we will be making trip plans to return, even before we head home.

Here's my rationalization for all this traveling for my treatments. It's only a 10 hour flight from here. If treatments like this were available in North Carolina, we would be driving 12 hours without even questioning it. If I just pretend the flight is a "drive", it's not so bad. So, we have to come to Germany a few more times. Life could be worse! In addition, each time we come, the weather will be a little different. There was snow this time, next time, flowers, then, more flowers with leaves on the trees. It can only get nicer and more beautiful here!

Saturday, March 7, 2009 12:30 AM

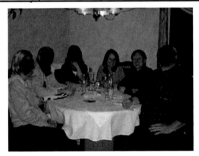

Summary of My Treatments Here

Guten Abend (Good evening) to all!

As you can imagine, we are very excited to be going home tomorrow. At times, it seemed as if this day would never arrive. We will miss our new friends we've made here. We hope to catch back up with them on a later trip. We will definitely be keeping in touch. Meeting them and becoming friends has helped tremendously in coping with being away from my home and my family and friends back there.

We all went to a Greek restaurant tonight for dinner (see picture). The main course for dinner at the clinic was bruschetta on toast... the dinners here are the lightest of the day so we decided to walk to this place. We had a great time. Chuck of course, gave the waitress a silly hard time right from the moment we sat down until we paid our bill, which we didn't have enough cash for. Very few places accept credit cards here. Thank goodness for David, or 4 of us might have been washing dishes. The waitress was a really good sport through it all!

The walk to the restaurant led us through a big park with huge trees and winding paths behind the klinik. It was quite pleasant. It was daylight on the way there, but had gotten very dark for the way back. Up and down hills and around corners, with the moon shining through the trees. It would have been scary if there weren't six of us. It was actually very serene, and peaceful, and beautiful….. We made it back safely, although not the same way we went... wonder how that happened... certainly we didn't get..... LOST?

In the morning, I will be getting two more infusions "for the road", and then my infusion line will be pulled. Yep, a little nervous about that one. As a nurse, I really am a big baby..... The nurses here all understand. Most are the same way. Definition of nurse: picky, stickler, perfectionist, questioning everything, big baby!

I would like to summarize my treatments and therapies from the last 3 weeks "for the record".

- Immediate preparations upon arrival for Whole Body Hyperthermia including Detoxing with high dose intravenous vitamin C, 7.5 grams, and vitamins B6, B12, and Folate infusions for 3 days.

- Blood tests are performed for white blood cells, red blood cells, platelets, and thyroid function as well as any others the doctor deems necessary.

- Electrocardiogram to check the heart's function and Lung Function Test to screen the health of the lungs.

- Local hyperthermia - lasting 1 hour each time is started right away and continued each day except on Sundays – only infusions are given that day. A full explanation of this treatment is on pg. 12.

- Oxygen Therapy - 2 liters of oxygen per minute during local hyperthermia. This therapy increases oxygen in the body. Cancer cells don't like oxygen.

- Foot and back massages. They really are a detoxifier...... Really!....(each, twice per week) More if you cry a lot from being homesick. Message moves stagnate lymph fluid out of the tissues for excretion from the body.

- Magnetic Field Therapy for 20 minutes followed by an ozone injection - twice per week. This therapy helps realign the magnetic pull possessed by all cells in the body thereby increasing effectiveness of certain treatments and reducing any pain. There is no "unusual feeling" during this treatment.

- Whole Body Hyperthermia with low-dose chemo. The core body temperature is slowly raised to as high as your body can tolerate, up to 107.8 degrees F. They raised mine up to 105.8, which Dr. Herzog was very pleased about. At that time, the temp was maintained for one hour, during which the low-dose chemo was infused. They used numerous medical monitoring methods, all of which I was very familiar with, which helped me realize it was a safe and professionally run procedure!

  One of the chemo drugs the doctor used for me, Mitomycin, becomes exponentially activated by heat to become much stronger. Normally it is a very weak chemo drug. Then, when the heat is gone, the strength comes down as well, hence the ability to have done major damage to "bad" cells without the massive damage to healthy cells.

The other drug he used, Vinorelbine, is a stronger drug to start with, but also becomes very damaging to the "bad" cells when heated. In this way, the whole body is treated as well as the specific areas of concern. After a cool-down period, they allow you to wake up – they infuse IV sedation during this treatment since it would be uncomfortable to be awake. Some have gone through it without sedation and they say it's very hot und uncomfortable.

Afterwards, I didn't remember a thing, I was just tired. After 2 hours in a recovery room, they wake you up for dinner then you go back to your room for a good night's sleep. A detox regimen is started the day after the low-dose kimo/whole body hyperthermia.

- After one week, during one of my local hyperthermia treatments, a repeat of only the Vinorelbine was given. The local hyperthermia treatments actually make a specific area hotter than it can become during "Whole Body" due to the fact that it's a small area being heated and not all the organs in your body. Again, the Vinorelbine combined with the heat becomes activated to kill "bad" cells with much more strength at a much lower dose. In addition, heat alone can kill "bad" cells, but combined with low-dose chemo just adds to the collateral damage to "bad" cells. A detox regimen is again started the day after the low-dose chemo/local hyperthermia.

- Here is a list of the detoxing and/or immune boosting infusions used for me: High dose intravenous vitamin C, vitamins B6, B12 and Folate, Selenium, Thymus extract, Lymphdiaral, Acetylcystein, Glutathione, L-Carnitine. All are natural and not chemical except the Selenium and vitamin C. When I got the bad cold he gave me Erkaltung's Cocktail, a natural cold remedy by infusion. I felt great in 3 days. Echinacea drops, by mouth, are used freely and daily for helping to increase the WBCs back to normal. For the little bit of queasiness and/or loss of appetite that occurs, Reglan liquid is given which really helped. If a stronger drug is needed for symptoms, more is available, but I did not need anything else.

It's been a very interesting journey and we've been very happy with the experience and treatments received from the clinic.

Wednesday, March 11, 2009 9:38 PM

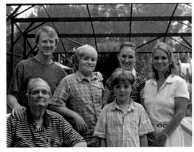

Burned at Home, Not in Germany!

We are back at home, finally! It is sooooo good to be home! You cannot imagine!!! I've been keeping busy the last few days at home with appointments and getting back into what I need to do around here. I'm definitely very busy.

I must have forgotten how to cook while away because I was absent minded in the kitchen and burned the heck out of my right hand and finger. As I lifted the lid off of a boiling pot of my special detox tea, hot steam spewed out directly onto my hand. The immense pain, blistering and redness told me it was a second degree burn, which is actually the most painful of burn types. The blister that occurred on my toe in Germany was nothing compared to this. I had my hand in cold icy water for hours before the pain began to subside just so I could do anything around here except sit with my hand in the water. Even typing was difficult, as I couldn't blow on my hand and type at the same time. The pain was barely tolerable as long as I kept dipping my hand in the ice water and blowing on it while writing.

For now, I will be adjusting to being back home and taking care of the family until it's time to leave again for Germany for another round. I feel great and have plenty of energy for riding bikes with my 2nd grader, and am enjoying the warmth of the sun back here in Florida.

One thing I've discovered with all this, is that it really takes a lot of time, effort, organization, and dedication to take good care of yourself when you don't have great lifestyle habits to begin with. The saying is true, "a stitch in time saves nine", meaning that since I spent so many years not taking great care of myself, now I have to put forth 9 times the effort to get well. A simple "stitch" to keep things healthy from the start would've saved all this from occurring.

We will only have to be in Germany for 10 or 11 days this time. That should be a lot easier! I want to give a huge thank you to my Aunt Frances for taking such amazing care of my family in our absence. She and my grandma are heading back to Alabama tomorrow morning and Chuck needed to go out of town on business. So, I will be on my own until he gets back on Friday night.... It's just a couple of days but there's a lot of readjusting after being gone so long. Thank you everyone for your continued support and prayers.

SECOND TRIP TO GERMANY

Sunday, March 22, 2009 11:27 PM

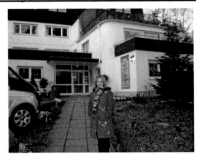

Round Two Begins

Everything went great at home and we had a wonderful time for the last 3 weeks being with our family and friends. However, the party must end and here we are again, back in Germany for a second round of treatments including local hyperthermia, one whole body hyperthermia, and another round of low-dose kimo. The plane was packed coming over here so we had to try and sleep sitting up in our seats. Needless to say, we didn't get much. When we got to the clinic it was immediately time for two IVs (vit C and vit B's), and straight to bed.

After a 4 hour nap, we had dinner, talked with friends we knew from before, and met new friends, already. We are off to bed again now for the rest of the night, thank goodness!

Monday, March 23, 2009 6:15 PM

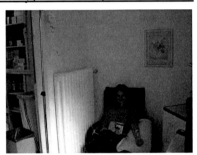

Back, with a PICC in My Arm

Guten Abend!

We're back in the swing of things already! It's a much easier adjustment the second time around. There is a lot going on here. The place is very busy with patients and I'm on my 4th infusion for the day. We met some wonderful new people as well as catching up with friends from before.

Our friends Lin and Sue, from church, came up the day after we left last time. Lin has liver cancer, spread to the lungs. This is their first visit here. Lin's doctor told him there was nothing that could be done for him in Florida so they decided to also come to Germany for his treatments. Just as we got back here, they were preparing to leave to go home, so we got to catch up with them. They are great and I hated to see them leave this morning after their 3 weeks here. Lin has a great attitude and seemed to be having way too much fun here... What's the deal with that????? I need some of that to rub off on me!

Back in Florida, I asked my holistic doctor to please order a specific IV line for my infusions in Germany so the "neck IV" wouldn't have to be re-inserted. If I had come back with nothing, they would have put a "needle in my neck" like last time (I really didn't like that). I requested what's called a PICC line, Percutaneous Intravenous Central Catheter. I had it inserted at a hospital in Florida, on Wednesday. It goes into a large, deep vein in the inner bicep area of the upper arm. From there, the catheter is threaded up the arm and around to the heart where the tip of it rests just outside the heart in the large vein there. This is a sterile procedure done with guidance by ultrasound by two specialized nurses. They were reassuring and knew exactly what they were doing. I was impressed with how quickly it was done. It wasn't much worse than getting a regular IV inserted because they numbed the area in the upper arm first. That's what hurts.

Typically, a port is surgically inserted in the upper chest for kimo drugs, which is what most of the patients have at the klinik. However, I chose not to get that done due to the possible complications that might have interfered with our trip back here this time. My fears are not unfounded. My own mother, upon her diagnosis of breast cancer, was scheduled to have a port inserted. The doctor accidentally punctured her lung which resulted in having to have two huge painful "chest tubes" inserted into her side for a few weeks. It made quite an impression on me. This is a very rare complication but I just needed to do something different. Also, I have seen many develop infections at their port sites. I hope the PICC line will be a success for my needs here.

The problem with the PICC line is, it doesn't infuse as fast as the "neck line" or a port, so I will need to have a regular IV in my arm for the large amounts of fluids given during Whole Body Hyperthermia (WBH). Having a needle inserted in my arm for that one day shouldn't be too bad. Maybe one day, needles won't bother me........wishful thinking!

Today I had an ultrasound of the breast/axilla area, local hyperthermia, ozone shot, magnetic therapy, and a back massage. We haven't even gone outside. It's cold and rainy and we even heard a clap of thunder tonight. That part made it feel like Florida.

Poor Chuck, he's here in the room trying to pry off the top of a non-alcoholic (translated, 2 and a half percent alcohol) lemon pilsner with a butter knife. That's not working, no surprise. Now, he is banging it on the lever handle of the bathroom door. Earlier, I had him running around getting me hot water, a spoon, a fork... you name it. I'm hooked to an IV so I'm helpless and have needs, what can I say?

We still have jetlag but I'm hoping to get some good rest when they "make" me sleep for the Whole Body Hyperthermia bright and early tomorrow morning... around 7:30. I guess Chuck will be glad I'm out of commission for a while. Then he can get some rest too.......... Wow, he actually got that bottle opened........ I'm impressed!

I'm thrilled that I was present to hear this personally. There was a guy named Tom from Canada we met last night. Canada's socialized healthcare is worse than our healthcare. If the government doesn't think you have good life expectancy based on the money they spend to get you well, they just quit treating you. Well, he came here with pancreatic cancer that spread to the liver and lung, 39 tumors in his liver alone! His doctors in Canada told him to go home and get his affairs in order. They refused to even try to treat him. Well, he came here instead. I got to see the big smile on his face last night when he came and announced that this was his last trip he needed. Dr. Herzog told him that the lung and liver tumors were gone and there were only a few minor issues in his pancreas, which will be treated and monitored at home. It is so encouraging to see this happen. There are many other stories here that we hear about, but I love seeing it with my own eyes.

This was in an email, a personalized Bible verse, sent to me from my sister in Chicago. It was much needed today. Thank you, Clarissa.

> *"Be strong and courageous, Laura. Do not fear or be in dread of them, for it is the LORD your God who goes with you. He will not leave Laura or forsake her." Deut 31:6.*

Tomorrow, already, I will be having my WBH and hopefully a report from the ultrasound taken this morning.

Tuesday, March 24, 2009 7:15 PM

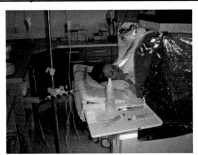

Improvement on Ultrasound!!

Hola Everyone! ("Hi" in Spanish - thought I would mix up countries tonight)

It was one of my favorite days... I got baked (Whole Body Hyperthermia-WBH). No Italian cheese, no chocolate chips, just me! How is this my favorite day you ask? Well, afterwards, I felt great but sleepy when I woke up. Then I got to sleep to my heart's content, food I requested was brought to me, and everyone was happy to see me up walking around and telling me how great I look. Even my hair got compliments! Of course, it was a great day! AND the whole day just flew by since I slept most of it. I'm coming home in 9 days! (pictured is me, totally out and dreaming I'm at the beach, ready for WBH. Then they kicked Chuck out of the room)

But wait, there's more!.... All this is working!.... At 11 pm last night, Dr. Herzog popped his head in our room to let me know the results of my ultrasound (he knew I was very anxious about it). Two of the three affected lymph nodes have shrunk to normal and the third is smaller! I give all the glory and praise to God for the healing He is giving!!!!!!!!!!!!!!!!!!!!!!! Thank you all for your prayers........ You have to be feeling the excitement in my "typing" voice.

Not that it matters at all, but I did get a few more surface burns than last time from the WBH. Front and back of lower legs. A toe on both feet and my left elbow. They don't hurt at all, but the nurses slather ICE COLD silver sulfodene cream and gauze all over any red spots after WBH while the skin is still very warm and cover with white fishnet. Boy, am I attractive.

My core temp got up to 105.44 F this time, which Dr. Herzog was happy with. Last time was 105.8 F. It's a very unpredictable thing how your body chooses how hot it wants to allow itself to become, and where and how many skin burns occur. There's no rhyme or reason to it. They have certain protocols they follow so as not to injure anyone in the process of healing... what a novel idea!!!!

Of course, my finger is still wrapped up from my own cooking abilities from 2 weeks ago at home. They don't do any kind of damage like that here, except to cells that are misbehaving! I did have that extra IV put in my arm for the almost 4 liters of fluids given during WBH, which one of my favorite nurses inserted AFTER she put the sleepy meds through my PICC line so I would be "out" when she did it. How smart! Her name is Nadine. We nicknamed her "Needles Nadine" or "Needleen" because she's very good with needle sticks. She is very mild mannered, sweet and cute and we got a laugh from her about the new names we call her now. She understands most English but not all. I was happy to see her in the room when I arrived for my WBH.

It's been a great day... a really great day!

Wednesday, March 25, 2009 11:45 PM

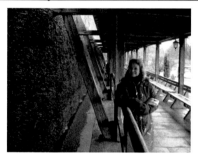

Jet-lagged, but Content

It snowed this morning... lots of big flakes! No snowman though, since the ground wasn't cold enough for it to stay. I just enjoyed watching it from our window. I have been soooo sleepy since having my Whole Body Hyperthermia (WBH) yesterday. We slept through breakfast, had to reschedule my 10 am massage and didn't get up until 11 am. It must be jet-lag because Chuck did not have WBH, that I know of, and he's just as tired.

Chuck and the nurses kept disturbing me all day, making me eat and other nonsense things like that! I just wanted to go back to bed. Chuck did manage to get me outside for the first time since we arrived on Sunday. We made it to the Lithium well for salty, metallic water... yum. That made it worth it? The weather is the usual frigid, wet like before but the fresh air did me well. I was more awake after that and the huge "salt producing contraption" in the park was working (see picture) so we hung around there a while and breathed in the healthy mineral-rich mist it produces.

Our bed is a little bigger than a twin so thank goodness I'm at my ideal weight (Wow, it's been a looong time since I've said that) That's what happens when you only eat what you're supposed to... who knew?

We have made another good friend, Jana, who is here with her 24 year old daughter, Jamie, who has a very rare form of cancer in her abdomen. There have only been 70 cases known. Her doctors in Texas had not dealt with it but Dr. Herzog has. I really like them. They are very upbeat and we have a lot in common with everything we have read and practiced regarding alternative treatments. Jamie looks fabulous and is engaged to be married. This is her 2nd trip here also.

It's very crowded here this week. Antje, my nurse, took all the gauze off my legs and left elbow and toes where I was "burned". I think they just enjoyed slathering that ice cold cream on me for fun because there were no burns except on the front of my shins and that 2nd toe, like before... Yeah, that was the worst part of my WBH day! I asked her how many patients were being seen because the staff seemed so busy. She said there were 36 patients being seen and there are 31 beds! Some stay across the street at the hotel. Word must be getting out about this place. Wonderful!

There are quite a few young couples here and everyone pretty much looks great. It's almost like a fraternity house with all the laughter and craziness, but no "kegs" to be seen, only Volvic waters, coffee and healing teas! Wow, we leave a week from tomorrow.... wow! I'm doing so much better this time. The first couple of days were rough with watching Lin and Sue leave, but the familiarity of people, and the shorter time period here... has made the transition much easier. But, I still require comforting words from home, though. I have a 10:00 appt in the morning so I really should be getting ready for bed. It's almost midnight now. Sleep is extremely important for healing.

Thursday, March 26, 2009 12:45 AM

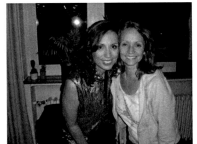

Beautiful Hungarian Opera Singer

First of all, thank you again so much for all the encouragement, prayers, online hugs and "drivebys" to check on my family! Hearing from home is my "lifeline". I look forward to reading the online letters every day and I hang onto every word.

Today was cloudy and cold with rain on and off again. Where is SPRING????? I felt pretty good this morning but meals got more difficult as the day progressed. I felt fine until it was time to smell food or eat. Again, kind of like a "morning sickness" feeling. It's 2 days after my low-dose kimo and this is what seems to happen. Great, this is what may happen next Thursday coming home after getting my 2nd dose on Tues. Maybe if I use the airplane sickness bag, someone will find me an extra seat to spread out on...ha! Have nausea meds, will travel!!!!!

I had 3 infusions today. L-Carnitine, which causes fat to be used for energy instead of muscle (don't you all wish you had some), Selenase (selenium) for decreasing side effects of kimo, and Lymphdiaral, a lymph detoxifier. Also, the usual magnetic field and ozone injection. I even fell asleep during my local hyperthermia. I "worked in" a back massage that should've been on my schedule... now listen, don't take away my massages!!!

We met with some new friends and went for a long walk. They are from Texas. This is their first visit here so we showed them around town a little. It was very refreshing outside with no food smells! Tonight after a dinner of toast, crackers, and pretzels (which were very good by the way), there was a concert with a professional opera singer in the lounge. Her voice was crystal clear, strong and beautiful! She is from Hungary (see picture). She sang songs like "Someday My Prince Will Come", "The Rose" (made me cry), "My God" from the movie Sister Act, "Ava Maria", a song from Phantom of the Opera, "Don't Cry for me Argentina", and the last one was "Time to Say Goodbye from Romeo and Juliet".

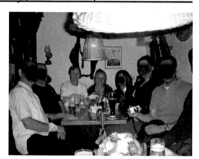

Definitely made me cry because that was one of the songs played by the "Winter Park High School, Sound of the Wildcats, Marching Band" all this year during which we volunteered many times. Morgan would have loved to hear her sing it. It was beautiful. She sang it in Italian. It really made me homesick for those fun days and how the marching band played it so beautifully!!!!

Moving on, after that emotional performance, one of the guys put on a video of a comedian named Russell Peterson...very funny. Even Antje, my nurse, came and sat for a moment to watch. She said her English isn't good enough for her to understand it though. She told me she needed to change my "bondage" (the way she says bandage), so I had to make sure she knew that bondage is not the same as bandage. She thought that was funny. She's so cute. We better get to bed. It's almost 1 am right now. I pray that all is going well for each of you at home!!!!

Friday, March 27, 2009 12:45 AM

Dagmar and the IV

I am so glad each and every one of you at home are in my life! Thank you for the notes and letters! A song I forgot to include that the singer performed last night has been stuck in my head all day. I just have to tell you what it is because she sang it so beautifully. It was from "My Fair Lady", "I could have Danced all Night"... great song!!!! She sang just as pretty as Audrey Hepburn, only louder. Chills!

This morning, I did not get out of bed until 12:30 because I knew my stomach wasn't ready to eat and I knew I wanted to sleep! I had a quick lunch then went for my massage.... real nice today. "Don't hate me because I'm being spoiled"!

I had 5 infusions today! L-Carnitine like yesterday, Thymus extract for immunity, Lymphdiaral for lymph drainage activity, Glutathione with N-Acetylcystein (NAC) a major immune booster for all cells, and calcium for my, again, cramping feet along with oral magnesium (one dose is all it takes and no more "charlie horse" feet). This happened after my last WBH treatment, too.

A funny thing happened with my IV today. Dagmar, your typical abrupt German nurse who eventually shows her compassionate inner self, does not like my PICC line. She's not familiar with it. Also, it runs slowly unless it's on a pump, which they don't do here like at the hospital at home. Anyway, I was getting impatient waiting for my IV to finish, so Chuck and I "rigged up" a tourniquet with a pen, tape, and my extra fishnet stocking tied around my IV bag to "squeeze" it to run faster. It actually worked great by the way. So, who walks into our room but Dagmar! She looked at it and just shook her head, mumbled something in German and turned around and left. She was the only one that I didn't want coming in at this time... and she rarely comes into my room.... Murphy's law! Chuck and I had a good laugh about that.......... after she left.

I had to convince the nurses to use both lines in my PICC so I could receive two IVs simultaneously. That's what they're there for! They checked with Dr. Herzog and he said "Yes, of course". Yep, I'm a typical nurse patient! Well, I can't be sitting here getting infusions for hours on end!

Tonight we had such a good time after dinner. About 12 of us went to a little pub down the street (see picture). Very quaint authentic German pub. Our half was the rowdy end of the table. I brought my resveratrol drops (immune boosting ingredient in red wine but no alcohol) to add to "still" water (no bubbles) so I could have a nice, very healthy sipping drink that looked like wine. After about an hour, one of the traveling male nurses from the klinik met with us there and he was just as rowdy. There were jokes, cheers, getting to know one another and lots of laughing. We sure livened up the place with our loud laughter. Waters and fassbiers (draft beers) cost the same... 2 euros.

I'm surprised, but my stomach is already feeling a lot better tonight and I had a nice sized dinner. Whoever prayed for that, or even thought about praying for that......... THANKS! We come home in 6 days.... YAAAAAAAY.... Wait a minute, I'll have to cook, clean, get up early..... hmmmmm. Oh, who cares, I can't wait to get home!

Saturday, March 28, 2009 10:20 PM

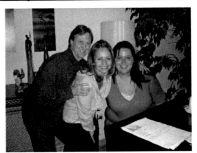

Concert by Andrea

Today has been a "tired" day, again. I tried to convince Chuck that they turned me into a half-vampire (sleeping all day) when they put that needle in my neck last time. He didn't go for it. Then I tried to tell him I was trying to break a World Record and I had to stay in bed or it would invalidate my efforts. He didn't go for that either. He made me get up and eat and shower! Such torture! After all, it was only noon, or 1, or something like that.

Dr. Herzog came in to see us and put me on something else, for energy. He is also big into Sports Medicine and is head of a long distance bike riding team. He gave me "Anabol-Logus", a natural supplement that helps people recover from marathons and such, quicker, and helps prevent muscle tightness and fatigue. It was even used by one of the Olympic teams, legally. I don't know if it can be purchased at home but is available on the internet. It can take the place of NSAIDS at preventing muscle pain after exercising... I'll give it a try!

The time changes here tonight, "spring ahead", so we'll be back to 6 hours difference from home again instead of 5. We've turned our clocks ahead already so we can try and get to bed at a decent time. That's hard when you're a "vampire".

They did another ultrasound on my neck this afternoon because Dr. Herzog forgot to look there a few days ago. Everything is the same there as before...no noticeable lymph nodes, i.e., "no spreading". I didn't expect any but was still nervous nonetheless. My local hyperthermia was during dinner so I just got a quick peanut butter and banana sandwich and grapefruit, which is exactly what I needed. My stomach still isn't back to normal yet and I've lost 3 kilograms, about 6 pounds. I'll put it back on like last time. I still look good and feel good except the smells of the foods just make me queasy right now.

This afternoon we were treated to a 45 minute mini-concert from one of the patient's daughters (see picture). She played piano and sang some soft music from artists like Elvis, Michael Buble', and two songs she herself wrote. Her name is Andrea and she is from Canada. She was in "Canadian Idol" (like America Idol) and came in 48th, which is phenomenal. She sounded fabulous. We all loved it so much that she said she will do a couple of these next week. It was nice to see when someone who is so young had found her niche.

Later we went down to the gym for some mini-trampoline bouncing and a few intense yoga moves. Chuck twirled a staff and kicked the punching bag a few times. We found a radio with Bon Jovi on the station. They sure like American music here even though they don't understand the meaning, or the words, most of the time.

I'm working on my 3rd out of 4 infusions for today. They started them this evening during local hyperthermia. They only have one nurse on duty at night. Antje is here! She's letting me hang my 4th infusion myself. I don't think the other ones would have let me do that even though it's not a big deal. Today I'm getting Calcium, L-Carnitine, Selenium, and Lymphdiaral.

Sunday, March 29, 2009 10:15 PM

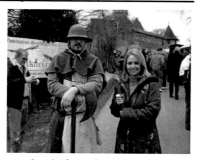

Medieval Easter Market Trip

The klinik arranged a trip to a medieval castle in Ronneburg for the Easter Market today (see picture). I'm so excited and two van loads will be going. Sundays around here are the slowest day of the week with only infusions and I had 3 this morning. After Chuck made me eat lunch it was time to leave for the castle. Two, crowded but fun, van loads from here (Dr. Herzog's treat) traveled about 35 minutes to get there. As we traveled up a winding road and rounded a corner in the van, we could see a huge, real-life castle up on a hill surrounded by huge trees and vast areas of land with people dressed in medieval costumes selling their medieval "wares" outside. They were also in costumes selling food and items inside throughout the entire castle. The walls were thick and the towers were tall. We walked so many stairs to get around and took tons of pictures. There was even an indoor well that was so deep it took a full 10 seconds for water poured in at the top to hit the water at the bottom. You could barely even see the bottom even with strong lighting they had in it. It was so far away the bottom looked as small as a quarter even though the opening of the well was about 8 feet wide!

Vendors in authentic outfits were selling authentic Knight parts and weapons (expensive), medieval clothing, toys, food.....it was so much fun. Tons of people "dressed and acting the part" made it feel like we had gone back centuries in time. There were even sword fights! Of course, we got a few items for the kids.

My stomach is feeling a little better this evening, finally. We just got off from video conferencing with the family at home. Everyone looks great but they are missing us as we are missing them! Four days to home!

Detoxing Pep Talk and Information

This evening, I would like to emphasize the importance of "detoxing". This is something I hadn't participated in before. You hear about it, maybe, but it's not something you'd see on a TV ad, so most people don't think it's important.... it's IMPORTANT! That is what half the infusions are about that I am receiving.

And the more I learn, from all that I have been reading and researching, detoxing is like caring for your car. You would never, ever run your car for years without changing the oil or getting a tune-up! Why do we abuse our bodies as such when each day we are bombarded by toxins in the air, water and foods we consume! Or even stress!!!!! Lest our bodies become stagnant and very vulnerable to all kinds of illnesses and diseases, we must detox!

Detoxing should be done in a particular order and several times per year, just like an oil change. I wish I had known about this a long time ago!!!! I learned it's of utmost importance to be patient and not rush through detoxing as it is like peeling away the layers of an onion, whereas if you go too quickly you can experience uncomfortable symptoms as the toxins are trying to leave the body.

In the process of detoxing, there are "toxins" trying to exit at the same time which can put a strain on different organs, such as the liver and kidneys. This is why only one organ should be cleaned at a time, starting with the bowels (sorry, I had to say that word), then kidneys, then liver and gallbladder (especially if your gallbladder has been removed). Did you know that gallbladders have a very important function and with detoxing, removal of them is totally avoidable... who knew????????????? Please go to any health food store and ask them for their "expert" on detoxing and spend some money on your health NOW.

Chuck has decided to start "changing his oil" as soon as we get home from our trip here. I have "people" helping me with this so don't think all this is MY idea! I'm still learning, but at a Mach V rate, because of this "challenge" I'm facing head-on!

Just one more note on detoxing. Any of you ever wake up in the middle of the night with anxiety and worry and can't go back to sleep? I used to do that about 4-5 times per week. Even with this challenge I am dealing with, since I've been getting detoxed, I have not woken up even one night feeling that way, for several months! For the first time in YEARS, I have been sleeping soundly through the night with NO medications whatsoever.... I am amazed at that!

Monday, March 30, 2009 11:45 PM

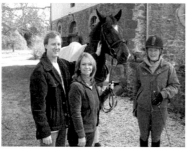

Shopping in Giessen

Whoa, where did the time go today. Actually, it's so late it's now.....Tuesday. But this is my Monday writing. Real quick since I have a 9 am appt. We had a very enjoyable day today going to Giessen, a bigger city for shopping about 30 minutes away, with another couple from Australia. This evening was spent in the lounge at the klinik sharing funny stories. There was the couple we went with today, along with another couple from South Africa. We discovered how our kids have similar quirks and are really the same no matter where they are raised. We all have so much in common even though we are from different corners of the globe! It's so good to be able to laugh so much here! Something about it makes my stomach feel better.

Chuck had some work to do tonight, which is a good thing, but I was not able to get on the computer to write until very late. I must get to bed since it's 1:35 am now and I am due to receive a low-dose kimo treatment tomorrow so am asking for exxxtra prayer for protection and healing. It will be at 3:30 my time so 9:30 in the morning for most of you. I love you all!!

Tuesday, March 31, 2009 11:45 PM

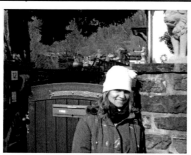

The problem with Socialist Medicine and Another Musical Concert by Andrea

Starting with tonight, we were again treated to another musical concert in the lounge by Andrea Gal (she is pictured with us on the March 28 entry) I enjoy her music more each time I hear her. She has so much talent and creative abilities. Andrea sounds a lot like Colbie Caillat who sings "Bubbly", which Andrea sang tonight. She writes half her songs which are fabulous, touching, and inspiring. I feel so blessed having her here and will miss her when we leave on Thursday.

Andrea is a strong, young, and beautiful person to be around. She is "genuine". I also would like to include her website so you can listen to excerpts from her songs and purchase CD's, if you'd like. It's www.andreagal.ca. One of the CDs is love songs and the other is Christian music. I bought them both. Her family just lost her dad from an aneurysm in January and now her mom is ill with a colon mass. The family flew her mom here to Germany from Canada via air ambulance because the airlines said she was too sick to fly with them. Don't even try to ponder the cost of that!

Her mom is Clara and she is just as sweet and strong. They are also here at the klinik, as socialist medicine in Canada had decided she was too expensive medically and refused to continue to treat her cancer. At least that's something they don't do in the U.S. They advised her to go home and get her affairs in order. Whether that's going to be the case or not, that should not be the decision of the government. I pray for the best for them.

Today I only had my ozone injection and then a pre-kimo infusion with cortisone, an anti-inflammatory, and two other drugs that lessen the effects on the stomach lining, and a nausea med, then the "low-dose kimo" during local hyperthermia. I prayed over the "pac-man medicine", then Chuck prayed over the "pac-man medicine". Thank you Pat, for that "visual" to concentrate on! Pac-man "eating" bad cells.........

We are praying for a comfortable and safe flight home on Thursday. The stomach queasiness usually starts in 2 days... Thursday, of course. I will ask for an infusion for nausea (which will be prayed over) that morning whether I need it or not. I also have some "drops" they give for nausea, which will be in my carry-on.

Today was sunny without a cloud in the sky! Gorgeous. I didn't get out for very long with the timing of my infusions, keeping me running up and down the stairs to talk with nurses and starting my infusions early enough so that the kimo was halfway done before my hyperthermia started. Remember my PICC line runs slow but I don't care, it's not in my NECK!

This evening at 11 pm I popped my head outside the clinic. The moon and stars were beautiful and it wasn't nearly as cold. It is so amazingly quiet here at night. No cars off in the distance, no people talking, no dogs barking... nothing but maybe the rustle of the leaves if there's a slight breeze. I have never heard such quiet nights in my life. Not even with camping in the middle of the Ocala Forest in Florida! And the birds sing all day long as if it were morning! They love it here.

Tomorrow........OUR LAST DAY BEFORE GOING HOME!

Wednesday, April 1, 2009 11:00 PM

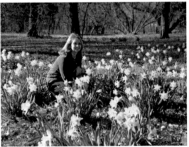

Tell Me Once Again!

Well, this is our last night here.....and that's not an April Fools joke! We met with Dr. Herzog with a list of questions. He answered them all and again we asked him if he was happy with the results of my ultrasound last week. He smiled and said yes, he was very pleased. He said there was a 200% decrease in the size and amount of the 3 visible lymph nodes, with 2 of them un-noticeable now and one reduced to half the size. We just wanted to hear his opinion again. It's nice to see a big smile as he says those results. He is a very quiet and caring person.

Last night I was in the physiotherapy area looking for a towel to go with my heating pad, which I use each night with my "castor oil pack". As I mentioned before, it's a treatment I apply to my right abdomen each night for liver detoxing. I came across a homeopathic cream called Lymphdiaral, which is the same name as one of my infusions here meant for increasing drainage in the lymph nodes. Well, I thought hey, I might be able to get some of that to bring home. Everyone could use more lymph node drainage. So, I asked Dr. Herzog about it and he said yes, I can get some sent from the pharmacy along with some other supplements we talked about.

He doesn't agree with everything we suggest but if you suggest something and he feels it may help, he goes for it. I like that about him. He's not stuck in his own little "box" of stuff. I also asked him for an extra ozone shot for today and he said yes to that. What the heck, load me up!

Tomorrow morning I'm getting some infusions and one more local hyperthermia "for the road". For the trip home, I have 2 anti-nausea liquids and will be getting another infusion for nausea. I haven't needed it but with altitude and turbulence, it won't hurt to get a little something extra. My blood work was done today and seems to be holding up. My red blood cells are a little low but everything else is great. I'll be having it tested again in a few days at home. Strange, no problems with white blood cells and platelets this time. Now I need to eat for the "red". More information to pull from the recesses of my "nurse brain". I remember something about raisins... or I can just look it up on the internet!

This afternoon the weather was just gorgeous. I sat in the sun on the patio for about an hour while Chuck got a massage. They only charge 6.50 euros for a half-hour full massage, not a chair massage! That's less than $10! Then he went to pay for it and the receptionist just said "aghhh" and waved her hand... that means "no charge". Of course, he had just paid the hospital bill so she probably felt he needed a free massage! Then Chuck and I went for a long power walk in the park to enjoy the warmth, probably mid 60s in the sun, and the flowers that have been popping out of the ground (see picture) as well as tons of freshly planted pansies. We drank Lithium water and just enjoyed the fresh sunny air! Nice! I will miss my new friends here (we've exchanged emails). We will see most of them next time around, but as Dorothy says it best "There's no place like home!"

Friday, April 3, 2009 6:00 PM

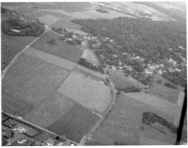

Rough Plane Ride but Home at Last

We made it home safely! This trip in Germany was definitely quicker and I didn't cry nearly as much from homesickness.... key word, "nearly".

I feel like I'm living someone else's life or reading a story about someone else. It's hard to believe, I am the story. It's all been so surreal. I also don't "feel" like I'm out of the woods yet and am keeping my guard up even though the Dr. tells me how good things are going. Knowing me, I will probably always keep my guard up. I don't know if that's a good thing. I hope to one day soon, be able to feel totally peaceful about my health. That's one of my major prayers and Bible study I've been working on. I need to feel peaceful in order to enjoy life and relax.

The flights to and from Germany have been fine for the most part...some rough air and a dip, causing a "roller coaster" effect, coming from Germany, enough that all 180 people on board went "woooo" and then you could hear giggles coming from everywhere. The landing was rough too, so much that everyone started clapping when the flight attendant announced our arrival at the Cincinnati Airport! There was a lot of turbulence from Cincinnati which cleared 15 minutes before we landed.....it figures! We had a 6 hour layover in Cincinnati which was long but relaxing. We found some comfortable seating at Starbuck's for a couple of hours and ate snacks here and there.

It was actually our 20 year anniversary yesterday so we had an extra 6 hours as we turned back the clock on our way home! Since we were practically there already, I could have gone to Paris or Italy to celebrate, and put off coming home, but I really just wanted to come home.

It feels strange, my body thinking it's almost midnight right now and being awake for over 24 hours yesterday... catnaps on the plane don't count a whole lot for sleeping. But overall I feel great. My stomach did amazing with all that turbulence, thank you God! I thought my stomach was back to normal until Chuck heated up a leftover casserole earlier... ugh. I had to shoo him away because of the smells. I do great with foods that don't put off a smell while they're cooking. This morning I had toast with honey and cinnamon, some egg salad that Aunt Mary made... yum, and lots of frozen berries, yum! The queasiness should only last another day or two.

Heading out for a quick bike ride with the boys, then we are off to Wal-Mart so they can spend their allowance. It feels so good to have some normalcy back, and to be home again!!!!!!!!!!!!!!!!! We're scheduled to head back to Germany.........April 21. I know, it's soon, but definitely important. Again, we just tighten our belts and do what we need to do!!!!!!!!!!!!!!

Third Trip To Germany

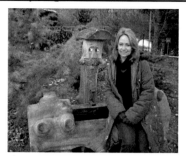

Positive News for Others, Too!

We made it to Germany safe and sound once again. An uneventful plane trip. Just a few bumps and such, nothing out of the ordinary. Crowded as normal... and not able to sleep well sitting up, so we are still up from when we left yesterday with only a couple of cat naps here and there... On the plane, we watched the movie "Yes, Man". It was quite thought provoking. Jim Carrey was his usual comical guy making me laugh for the duration of the movie. I also read a lot of my "positive thinking" books and we ate. Not much else to do on a long flight.

What's very strange about the trips over to Germany is that on the plane, at about midnight according to my watch, they start serving breakfast. Looking out the window, you begin to see the morning light appearing for the day. Then, you turn your watch ahead 6 hours. So midnight now becomes 6 am. Your eyes see it, but your body doesn't agree! The confused stomach and the fuzzy brain are in full effect for our first day here.

We are in a different wing of the klinik this time and had trouble getting the internet going. Also, there is a beautiful flowering tree right outside our sliding door... that's good, that has bees all over it... that's bad (see picture on April 22 entry). They have found a way into our room about 6 times today even with the sliding door closed. We want to open it for the fresh air but there is no screen. We'll talk to the handyman here tomorrow about all that. Our room has two twin beds, one of which is a hospital bed. I'm not sleeping in that! I'm not sick! It's also way over there on the other side of the room from the other bed. I'm not sleeping by myself either. Sooo, Chuck and I will be sleeping in one twin bed. We'll see how that goes. What can I say? I feel very needy right now.

One of our friends here will be leaving on Friday and we are going to try and nab their room downstairs. It's as big as our living room with 1 and a half baths! This one is like a hallway with two nooks, but we do have a great view of the beautiful tree and live bee entertainment!

Even though this is our first day here, I've already had my vitamin C and B's infusions, Magnetic Therapy, Ozone injection, and Local Hyperthermia. One of the doctors just finished seeing us and going over initial plans, nothing out of the ordinary. We'll see Dr. Herzog for more info and maybe an ultrasound tomorrow??? He's the one to talk to. They are very busy here with patients "squishing out of the walls". Word is getting out! This is the place to be!

I spoke to a few of my new friends from here and got some great news from them. One woman was told by Dr. Herzog that her cancer is gone. It was breast and lymph nodes and a tumor near there somewhere. Another friend had 2 MRIs and a CAT scan in Texas and only has some liquid filled cysts left which are not cancer, so Dr. Herzog said she is fine now also. Hers was breast, lymph nodes, and some cancer cells in the fluid outside her lungs, and they thought it had spread to her ovaries according to previous tests. All these are encouraging to me and I love hearing these stories.

With the busy-ness out of the way, we hope to catch up on some much needed sleep.

Wednesday, April 22, 2009 10:00 PM

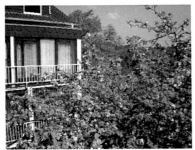

A German Liver Cancer Treatment

Today's treatments: vitamin C, B, and Thymus extract infusions, magnetic therapy and ozone shot, local hyperthermia, ultrasound (no results yet), and foot massage (nice!). Today I'm feeling a little more rested. I guess I don't move too much at night because sleeping double in a twin bed didn't bother me at all. Chuck may have something different to say about that though.

Looks like we'll be staying in this room after all. I'm looking at all the positives about it. The tree outside our sliding door is beautiful with solid white flowers. We are at the end of a hallway so it's very quiet. And they put up a screen today so only 2 bees got in. I'm getting used to them and it's only during the day. They're just looking for a place to make honey, not like on the movie "Killer Bees". They don't bother or sting us. Also, I'm near the nurses room so now I can bug the heck out of them "in person" instead of on the phone.

We learned of another interesting procedure they do in Germany, and not in the U.S. It is for liver cancer. There are 2 men here having it done. They go to a Frankfurt hospital and a catheter is inserted into the vein in the groin, and threaded up to the liver where kimo is injected directly to the tumor. This is done several times until the tumor has shrunk to a certain size. Then they go back and have a laser surgery done to obliterate what's left of it.....cool. There are less side effects and more concentrated kimo right where it's needed.

Tomorrow I'll be getting my Whole Body Hyperthermia (WBH) so pray that everything goes perfectly and that the low-dose kimo does a "well done" job, but that I come out rather "medium well".

It makes me feel a little closer to home that one of the guys here has been walking around in this bright blue jogging outfit with "Gators" written in bright orange on the sleeves. Hmmmm, wonder who he cheers for at football games? He and his wife live in Gainesville, Florida (home of the gators football team) and today is his 66th birthday. He had cake and flowers that were sent from friends in Texas (well, I'm sure they actually came from here because the cake and flowers looked much better than we did getting off the plane from the U.S.). I had a very small sliver of cake. They don't put a lot of sugar in their goodies here. It was splendid! A spongy yellow cake with ample whipped cream frosting. Afterwards, we went for a brisk walk and saw lots of exquisite flowers, and the trees have glorious green leaves, finally.

I can't end this entry without saying how much I miss everyone at home and I'm hoping that the next few days go by much faster. It's always a slow start when we get here. The first few days seem to drag even though I'm so busy. I guess I'm just adjusting, that's why I like my WBH day. They put me to sleep, then afterwards I just sleep the day away. It goes by quickly, and I'm not supposed to take any supplements that day.... it's a vacation from taking all those pills. I'm doing a lot of reading (positive Christian books). I crave them. Sometimes, just a paragraph is all I have time for. I make sure to have several reading choices at any one time to choose from, right now it's four. After all this, I should be the happiest, healthiest person on earth. What can I say? I'm practicing being positive and I do have a ways to go......

Thursday, April 23, 2009 10:00 PM

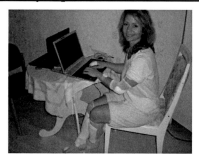

Chemo plus Typing = Frustration!

Post WBH. I'm up typing and making lots of mistakes. I guess even though I feel awake after the sedatives wear off, my brain is still "on drugs". My Whole Body Hyperthermia went well except I'm wondering why they only got my temp up to 104.4 F. The last two were 105.5 and 105.8. That's a question for Dr. Herzog when we see him next. They slathered that icy cold goop (silver nitrate cream) on every red area they could find on my legs.... burrrr! Back to the white fishnet stockings to hold all the gauze on (see picture).

That's it! I'm not typing anymore today! I'm normally about 50 words a minute with typing but this has taken forever with all the mistakes I'm having to fix.

Friday, April 24, 2009 10:00 PM

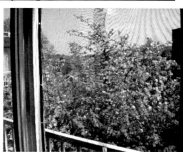

Germany vs. Mexico Cancer Treatments

Today's treatments were local hyperthermia, vitamin C and Bs, thymus injection, Magnetic Field and Ozone shot. Oh yeah, and a great back massage from Max. I took off the fishnet stockings this morning and only had a little redness remaining on my left shin from the WBH yesterday.

Today has been a tired day. I'm holding on to about 7 pounds of retained fluid as a result of my treatment yesterday. That's what usually happens but the scale is right down the hall now so it's easier for me to see just how much. That's almost a gallon! On the positive side, I actually look much younger since all that fluid makes any wrinkles less noticeable. People have commented on how great I look today. I guess retained fluid "becomes" me! It made walking up hills today somewhat "huffing and puffing". Ya'll strap a gallon of milk to your bodies and go jogging if you don't believe me!

Well, my ultrasound report was good again! That 3rd lymph node was 0.8 cm last trip. Now it is 0.5 cm and Dr. Herzog said it could even be just scar tissue but it's hard to tell without removing it, which we are not doing at this time. It started out at 2 cm so something good is going on. I'll be having an MRI mid-May to have a comparison with the original MRI done in Nov/Dec which should show a big change according to the ultrasounds.

The weather has been grand! Of course not warm like Florida, but we did get out walking with just a light jogging jacket on. This evening, I hear rain outside. The flowering trees are everywhere and lovely. Today was very sunny and I caught the lady from Wisconsin sunbathing her white skin. I hope she didn't get burned. I think she fell asleep out there.

We also met a couple from Scotland. They have been to Mexico for treatment and they really disliked it because they said everyone there got the same exact treatment, unlike here where each individual gets treatment tailored for him/her. They said they like it here the best.... good to hear!!! They can't even find an integrative/natural doctor in Scotland. At least we have a lot in the states. I really like the one that I've started to see.

Chuck got the chance to be a nurse today and changed my dressing on my IV line in my arm. It was a "sterile" change so there was a lot of instruction going on from me so that he didn't "contaminate the sterile field". He did a great job, but I didn't have any voice left afterwards, as my nurse friends can imagine.

We took a picture of the bee tree outside our window (see photo). Even though a screen was put up the bees still find their way in, but only one at a time, and then find their way back out. I don't mind them coming in ever since my friend Brenda said that maybe they are angels coming to visit me.

Saturday, April 25, 2009 11:30 PM

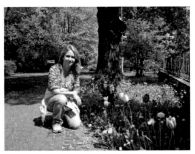

Fun Movie Night

We so enjoyed the outdoors and flowers and trees and birds today. The birds never "quiet up" until about 9:00 at night. They start at 5 am and don't stop or even let up! I've never heard such tweeting in my life.

After I finished my "stuff" by 12:30, we headed for Nidda, walking both ways, which we hadn't done before for some reason. We have usually taken the train either there, or back. We took some pictures of the flowers (check the tulips out) and views on the way. Everything is becoming so gorgeous here, very lush. A big difference from our first trip here when the trees looked like twigs and sticks and everything was gray.

In Nidda, I broke down and had...... PIZZA, for lunch. There were no lightning strikes so I suppose I'll survive the yummy ordeal. We walked a lot around the town and found a place to buy some organic nuts and dried fruit for the trip home.... yeah, it feels good to think about that! We planned to go to town with the couple from Wisconsin but he wasn't done with his "stuff" for the day so he couldn't leave yet.

Based on the MRI results I'll be getting at home, that I'll be bringing to Dr. Herzog next trip, we will determine what our next step will be. Here I am, two days post "kimo", walking 4 miles, and my stomach is pretty much doing ok, surprisingly. I'm taking the nausea drops since there was no appetite this morning. Just wanted to stay in bed.... but wait, that's normal for me. I always like to sleep in.

Tonight a bunch of us got together to watch the movie "Last Holiday" with Queen Latifah. It was very lighthearted and humorous. We all enjoyed it so much as we are all looking forward to a happy ending as well! Afterwards, the French lady (a patient here) was dancing around with her infusion bottle as if it were her dancing partner. She is so cut, fun, and loveable! Yesterday, while she was enjoying the peaceful quietude of the klinik grounds, smelling the flowers on the tree below our patio door, Chuck scared the heck out of her with a deep voice from above, "What are you doing?" If she needed an energy boost for the day, that did it! She took it very well and she started giggling after the initial scream and grabbing of her chest. She loves joking around but doesn't always expect Chuck's "out of nowhere" sense of humor. She does love it when people make her laugh.

When I had my massage yesterday, Max said I had a tight knot in my shoulder. Maybe it's from sleeping on half a twin bed. Do you realize how many inches that is? We'll see how much longer we can take that. The bees have become accustomed to our room. They are so amusing. They come in somewhere in the door jam and then promptly crawl out the opening slit in the screen, like it's a game. We thought we heard buzzing in the walls late last night.... honey anyone?

Oh yeah, back to why I'm here. My treatments today were local hyperthermia and two detox infusions - Selenium and Engystol. We started the magnesium tablets since we know that my feet get cramps after the kimo.

The glider plane was out for hours today, flying overhead and all around, the whole time we were out. I would love to take a ride in that thing. It's only out on the weekend and we don't know where its "home base" is. Tomorrow we get to sleep in since there is no "stuff" that goes on when it's Sunday except infusions. So it's ok that I'm up late tonight. We'll be looking forward to seeing Lin and Sue tomorrow as they return for his second treatment.

Sunday, April 26, 2009 10:30 PM

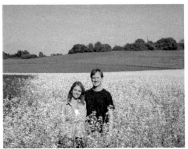

Eeek, My Nursing CEUs are Due!!!

We were glad to see our friends, Lin and Sue, get here safe from good ole' home to continue with his treatments. We spent time after dinner just chatting and catching up and talking about pizza and hot chocolate.

Today was a "work" day for me as I had to complete all my continuing education credits for my RN license before April 30th. Not unusual for me, I do this every 2 years when they are due. I just pulled the desk up to the window in the sun and worked for hours on the computer... got'er done! The day was so gorgeous and the birds were singing. It was actually easier doing them here with not much else to do, being Sunday... only infusions, Glutathione/N-Acetylcystein combo, and Lymphdiaral, both detoxers.

After that we went for a long walk in the park where a couple were on stage playing the keyboard and violin. One of the songs was "The Entertainer"....fun! We met up with a couple from the klinik and continued our walk. We took pictures of each other with the "oilseed rape plants", unbelievably bright yellow fields all over the place. (See picture) Hadn't seen that since Scotland 14 years ago. The fields are so bright you have to squint your eyes when you look at them.

On the way back, we stopped at a little cafe and had peppermint tea for me and red wine(rot wein) for Chuck. My stomach hasn't been too bad since my kimo on Thursday. I just don't like the smell of, or to think about, food. Right now I'm thoroughly enjoying strawberry granola, dried pineapple and almonds that we got from town yesterday ... organic of course. I suppose we'll need to get more for the trip home, teehee, which is what this was for.

Chuck just went to get me some German style "Boost", the nutrition drink for extra calories, and saw Dr. Herzog coming out of the office with a stack of files. He said he was going through them, reviewing them. He works such long hours and there are so many patients here. I worry about him. It's almost 11 pm here! Thank goodness another doctor rounded for him today. This seems to be his only day off and here he is working anyway.

We saw that glider plane flying around the park and klinik again ALL day long for like 8 hours. He's got to be giving rides to people. We've got to find out about that. I would love to go up in it.

<u>Monday, April 27, 2009 11:40 PM</u>

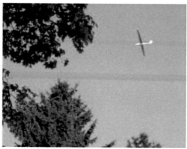

Birds, Birds, Everywhere!

Well, I'm up late again since we watched some French movie with English subtitles. I don't know the name. It was a true story about the writer/actor Molliere. It sure kept us on our toes, reading the subtitles the whole time. I may have even learned a few French words! Maybe...

Today we waited around the room for Dr. Herzog to see us. Then we could finally go to lunch. Afterwards, we headed out to the park with the lush hills behind the klinik. It was stunning out there. Everything was soooo green compared to last time and dandelions just cover the grassy areas. It felt like we were in Sherwood Forest with Robinhood. I really have never seen or heard so many birds in my life. Being German birds, I don't know any of their names. There was a large board with pictures, listing the many different kinds of birds. They were written in German, of course. It was fun exploring some new paths that we seemed to have missed last time.

I received 2 infusions - Selenium and Engystol, a detoxifier and an immune booster. My blood work is holding up ok. Nothing really bad. The numbers are down a little because of treatment last Thursday so they started me on Echinacea for the white blood cells, and the platelets are down some so I'm just trying to continue eating as healthy as I can. The Reglan (anti-nausea) has been really helping my stomach. It's fine unless I smell food, but am hoping it will be mostly back to normal tomorrow. The air in the klinik is fresher now that the weather is nicer and windows have been getting opened. Something about fresh air really perks up the stomach.

One of my favorite nurses, Antje, came busting through the door today and we squealed and hugged each other. She had been on vacation. We hadn't seen her since my last trip here. Her big smile just lights up any room!

A couple is leaving tomorrow for the last time. They are from Geneva. He had colon cancer (which was surgically removed in Vienna) that had spread to the liver, so they came here. He had local hyperthermias here and then Dr. Herzog sent him to Frankfurt for the special kimo liver perfusion followed by a laser knife procedure. This was his 3rd trip and Dr. Herzog said he only needs a check-up in 3 months. Another reassuring story.

It's raining outside right now and sounds so nice. It's also chilled up a little out there. We had to wear our coats in the park today. Speaking of all the birds I keep talking about, I want to share with you a verse that I read today in one of my positive books given by my sister-in-law, "Battle Field Of The Mind" by Joyce Meyer. It is from one of the many Bible verses about not worrying, from Matthew 6:26 – *"Look at the birds of the air; they neither sow nor reap nor gather into barns, and yet your heavenly Father keeps feeding them. Are you not worth much more than they?"*

By the way... so many friends commented on the glider I mentioned yesterday that I decided to put a picture of it with this entry. Maybe next trip we will see if we can get a ride.

Tuesday, April 28, 2009 11:45 PM

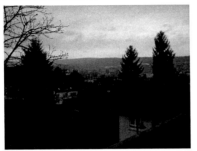

Local Hyperthermia Lesson

Today has been rainy and cold. I had the usual treatments, but Chuck got another back massage. I was present when a patient here needed to cancel hers so I jumped in and asked if Chuck could fill that spot. No problem, he really needed it!!!!

I fell asleep while trying to read and stayed sleeping for 2 hours. Also, I didn't get out of bed till 9:30 this morning. I need to stock up on this sleep for when I get home!!! We didn't get to go anywhere because of the rain, but finally couldn't stand being inside and we took a walk in the "hilly, woodsy, bird-filled" park for about 40 minutes. The fresh air was so brisk and.....fresh! Then we just hung out and socialized with friends in the lounge area. They had various beers they had bought today in town. I had water in a beer mug!

During our daily visit from Dr. Herzog, we asked him how the local hyperthermia machines in the U.S. differed from the ones used in Germany. He said the machines in Germany use "short waves" to generate the heat while the ones approved in the U.S. use "microwaves". Short waves have the advantage over microwaves in that they can penetrate up to 20 cm deep to treat cancerous areas in the body, while microwaves can only penetrate 3 to 7 cm. Also, local hyperthermia in the U.S. is not approved for use in conjunction with chemotherapy treatments (although clinical studies are underway). And that's a major reason why we are here.

Tomorrow morning starts early with a 7:40 am hyperthermia so I better get to sleep. Life at home needs to be more like this..... more sleeping and more socializing with friends and family.

Wednesday, April 29, 2009 10:00 PM

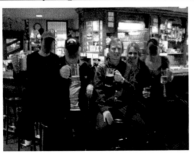

Walking in the Rain

For those who don't know when we are coming home.... it's this Saturday, May 2nd!!!! We'll be flying in at about 7 pm and my sweet friend and neighbor will be greeting us to take us home. It's earlier than usual due to a much shorter lay-over in Cincinnati. We will have to run to catch our connecting flight, which will not be a problem. I started early today at 7 for my local hyperthermia, then blood was taken, then breakfast, then a back massage, all done by 10 am. My ozone shot and Magnetic Field isn't until 1:30. The sun is trying to come out which we all really need today.

All the way over here in Germany, I read an article online that there is a case of Swine Flu at a hospital back home, from a Mexican traveler that was visiting one of the theme parks. Then, they were denying it until the CDC "confirms" it. Everybody, wash your hands constantly!

Also, I've been praying with Andrea, the beautiful singer/piano player from Canada. Her mom, Clara, needs our prayers at this time as well as Andrea. The doctor thinks Clara may be fighting an infection that is critical.

Even though it was cold and rainy today, we wanted to take the long hilly walk to Nidda for lots of fresh air and exercise. Chuck, Danny (a friend from the clinic) and I went even though it was raining. Chuck and I shared a very small umbrella. I kept, accidentally, hitting Chuck in the face with the umbrella so he decided to hold it instead (Pretty smart, aren't I).

After we got there, the rain let up. Once in town, we met with some more friends from the klinik, Richard and Sue, and went to a pub (see picture). I had bubbly water which "hit the spot" for my stomach We also got some more organic stuff for the trip home since we ate most of the other stuff we got for the trip. I got some food specifically to eat at the clinic since I REALLY needed some different, simple food. As soon as we headed back it started raining again. The air was crisp and actually enjoyable. We were well dressed with coats so were nice and warm.

I'm due for one of my low-dose kimo meds tomorrow, to be taken during my local hyperthermia treatment around 9 am your time. Please provide prayer for me that the kimo will do what it is intended to do and nothing else. My stomach is still not quite right. It's really not too bad though.

I would like to wish our wonderful friends, John and Pam, a Happy Anniversary on 20 years of marriage today!!!!!!!!!!!!!!!!!!

Thursday, April 30, 2009 11:45 PM

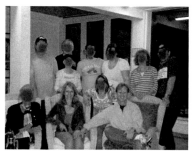

Being There for a Friend

I've had a tough few days here. Me, I'm fine, but Andrea's (the singer / songwriter / pianist) mom passed away last night. Andrea came to my room and we cried and prayed and laughed. It was very hard for me to do this with my personal experience I'm dealing with right now. I had to look past that and know that she was alone and should not be going through all this by herself. That would be a nightmare.

She came to our room at about 1 am last night and same the night before. She needed a friend and someone to help her know what was happening with all the IV's and everything. I was both of those for her and I'm glad I could be here for her. Yes, it was hard for me. I did not cry with her until after her mother passed away because I did not want her to be any more scared than she already was. THAT was REALLY hard. Of course, I cried back in my room and again first thing this morning as soon as I opened my eyes.

This evening, Dr. Herzog stopped me in the hall and thanked me for being there for her. I guess one of the nurses told him. He admitted it must have been hard for me with what I am going through. I thanked him for saying something. He's a compassionate person. Andrea's aunt came this morning and was a huge help for her. Her aunt is also a Christian.

For the rest of the day I have made myself busy socializing with anybody and everybody I could find. That made the day kind of fun! I even had the nurses laughing about a soda they were drinking in the office.... I saw it and the name was "Schlepp Schlapp", ok I know you just smiled, too. Every time I said it they just cracked up. German nurses really know how to laugh! That just caused me to include it in my sentences just so I could say it more. I thought it was odd that they laughed at it. They must be used to the name by now. But even when the nurse went to the room next door and heard me say it, she still cracked up laughing! What this drink is, is a cola/orange drink. I guess they never realized how funny it sounds when it's said with an "American" accent.

Of course, I had my low-dose kimo with the local hyperthermia and a massage... I did fine and feel great so far. I just have itchy earlobes.... I know, I'm strange. The same thing happened the last two times, so it seems to be "the norm"!

Chuck got to do some therapies today! He did it even though a "baby needle" was involved. I'm proud of him. With the Swine flu going around we decided to ask Dr. Herzog about some infusions for immune boosting for him since we will be flying internationally. He wrote Chuck a prescription without even batting an eye. I guess this is common here. Dr. Herzog's own dad is even here getting infusions to boost him up. He has some kind of heart trouble.

Chuck is getting vitamin C and Engystol infusions today, Friday and Saturday, then we leave. My alternative doctor in Orlando gives both of those instead of the flu shot.... interesting. Of course at home, the price is about 7 times more... here they will run about 30 Euros total each day (about 45 dollars) for the infusions, which includes administering them.... amazing, the prices here. Chuck also got a half hour massage from Max.... 6 euros, about 10 dollars! We're not talking a chair massage either. I had to talk Chuck into it since it was "Max" and not "Maxine". Max does a wonderful job working on those computer stress knots in the back and shoulders.

Tonight, a bunch of us got together for a pizza party in the common area. The party went on for hours. (See picture) Our friend from Munich, Vera de Winter, that helped set up the appointments with the klinik, arrived today so she joined the party as well. We chit-chatted and laughed and I even ate 2 very small pieces of pizza after dinner, which was steamed broccoli that the chef here made me (it tasted perfect!). I also had leftover pasta from yesterday's restaurant lunch, and before that, a pear and a kiwi. It really feels good to eat healthy all the time.

Friday, May 1, 2009 11:00 PM

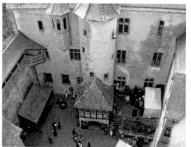

Dr. Herzog's "Giving" Heart

Our last night here, for now! We will be leaving in the morning at around 9 am, flying out at noon and arriving home around 7 pm. Of course, the actual time will be 6 hours longer than it appears to be, with the time difference.

We had a great day here. It's May 1st and a major Holiday here. You know, the Maypole thing? We didn't see any Maypoles though. We did go back to the same castle in Ronneburg, as during Easter time. It was a warm day and we got a couple of small things for the kids there. There was good food and entertainment and lots of stair climbing. That deep "well" there still fascinates me with how far down it goes!!!

Dr. Herzog sure has a big heart! We were all loaded up on the van to go and two more people came to get on. There were no more seats so another couple, obviously disappointed, got back off the van. Well, a little later, we saw them at the castle! I asked how they got here and they said Dr. Herzog found out about the van problem, got on his bike, and went and found them in the park. Then he arranged a driver to take them to the castle, and back. Yes, a big heart! And like last time, he paid for everyone to get into the castle/festivities. The day didn't cost us a thing except food and gifts!

Tomorrow morning will start early, around 6 am, since I will have about 3 or 4 infusions. I will be taking a preventive nausea infusion for the trip home, like last time. Also, I'm squeezing in one more local hyperthermia, then it's off to the airport. Can't wait to be busy at home giving hugs and kisses!

Again, we thank everyone at home for all the wonderful support, prayers, and entries you have provided for us! I want to put all this behind me, but know that I need to just "get through this storm" and I thank you all for helping us through it. It means so much more than you know! Every little bit helps, oh so much! I cannot wait for the opportunity to be on the "giving" side of helping others instead of the "receiving" side. I love each and every one of you!

Guten Nacht!

Friday, May 22, 2009 10:00 PM

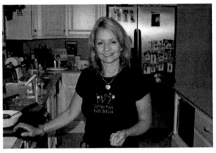

Back at Home and I Have Awesome Amazing News!

As I sit here drinking my carrot-apple juice..... I have news!!!!!!!!!!!!!!!! I had an MRI done on Monday and hadn't heard anything for a couple of days. I had Chuck call my doctor to get the results. I couldn't bear to hear anything bad. Nonchalantly, the doctor said "everything is fine", and they hung up the phone. Fine? What does "fine" mean? Everything's the same? Nothing's worse? I needed details!

I went to the imaging office the next morning, yesterday, and got the report, sat right there in the office, read it, and still had questions. I needed more details and to be able to understand all that I was reading. I'm a nurse and can read and understand most medical reports, and in the "impression", or summary, at the end of the report, it stated "Normal MRI". Normal for me? Or normal, normal? I needed to speak with someone right away! Calmly, I asked to speak with the radiologist who read my films, and a few minutes later they brought me back to her. My heart was pounding and it was hard to breathe.

She was wonderful with me. She sat me down in front of my films, which were displayed on the computer, and with excitement in her voice, proceeded to show me the comparisons. "There is no indication of any cancer on Monday's film." The results were normal! Everything that was there before, that was bad, is gone now. She turned to me and exclaimed, "What have you been doing?!!!

I told her, "a lot of alternative therapies and low-dose kimo". I didn't tell her about Germany yet. I just didn't feel comfortable going into the details with regular doctors about it yet since I've been keeping it under wraps for so long. Of course, through tears and laughing, I gave her a huge hug, and she said, "You need to be hugging someone else too. This is cause for celebration!" I will be giving Dr. Herzog that hug when we return to the klinik.

It was so wonderful seeing and hearing the excitement as she was showing me everything (now I'm crying again, tears of relief). She told me exactly what I needed, to settle my questions about it, once and for all. Then she said, "what now?" and I said I still have another dose of kimo to go and I'm not changing anything else or letting up on my therapies or regimens. She said "well, I guess I'll see you in like 6 months or a year!!!" She walked me to the front door and gave me her card and said don't hesitate to call if I have any other questions.

My breast surgeon here, wanted this radiologist to read my MRIs as she stated, "she is the best", so I feel confident in these findings. I have been thanking and praising God continuously. I'm not going to be like the 9 lepers that ran off happy and forgot to thank Jesus for their healing. He will hear it until He's sick of it..........

Even with these results we will still continue to follow the protocol set up by Dr. Herzog in Germany. It's kind of like antibiotics. You don't quit treatment just because things are looking well. You finish the whole treatment to prevent re-occurrence. We are leaving again for 12 days, this Sunday, on the 24th. I will be taking the new MRI results with me for Dr. Herzog to give his recommendations.

Thank you all so much for the prayers. Keep it up!

Fourth Trip To Germany

Monday, May 25, 2009 10:30 PM

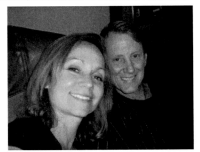

Woohoo, First Class!

We're back! In Germany, that is. First of all, we had the most amazing flight ever. It was odd how it came about. At home, Chuck wasn't able to print my ticket for some reason so we had to take care of it at the airport. Come to find out, somehow I had been placed as needing a wheelchair! WE did not do that and don't know how it got there. At the gate, when we went to get it straightened out, the lady noticed in the computer that we are "Medallion" status now (you know, with all the skymiles we've been racking up). She then asked us if we wanted 1st class even if we don't sit together......."Yes, duh". I didn't actually say that to her. So that was from Orlando to Cincinnati. Chuck ended up right behind me so we could still talk.

I had a chance to tell a man I was next to, about why I was coming to Germany. He works for Siemens and was also going to Frankfurt. He asked me why we were heading there so I very briefly gave him some key details about my treatments and how amazing the results have been. He seemed interested but I wasn't going to tell him too much unless he asked. He was, however, very happy for me. I did not want to go on and on unless he wanted to know more. I didn't want to be one of "those" people that talk the whole way when he had computer work to do. I suppose I planted a seed about German cancer treatment.

We had a pleasant, relaxing, 4 hour layover then it was time to get on the plane to Germany. A very nice lady behind the counter at the gate made some arrangements and we were bumped to 1st class, again!

This was the amazing trip. We walked in to Mimosa's and champagne being served followed by hot hand towels, 4 feet of legroom, chairs that recline fully, real pillows and blankets, warmed nuts in ceramic dishes, and a menu to choose dinner from (a 3 course meal). I had butternut squash ravioli, Chuck had Filet Mignon. I did splurge a little... "for the soul". After all, there was china, glasses, and real silverware. I was so beside myself I felt like doing a jig in the hallway. Chuck had to keep calming me down. I think I might have been embarrassing him. First a great MRI report, and then this!

I rested well but didn't really sleep soundly even though I was so very comfortable. In fact I was disappointed as we were getting close to landing. I told Chuck I was NOT leaving the plane. We also had Vanilla French Toast with eggs and orange juice for breakfast. Even if I never fly 1st class again, I am so grateful for the opportunity to have experienced this, and on an International flight!

Although quite jetlagged, I managed to spread the word at the clinic about my great report. The staff was all over me when we got here. After 10 minutes I was scheduled for my local hyperthermia, then Dr. Herzog came in and I told him right away about the MRI report and gave him that huge hug that I owed him, whether he liked it or not. I had a massage and the therapist also gave me a hug with hearing my news. I picked up my vitamin C and B infusions from the nurse and asked her about her pregnancy and told her my news. She was also very happy for me. I've been hugging people all day.

There are sooooo many people here this time that we know from previous trips. They are telling me how encouraged they are at hearing about my news. I am also hearing very encouraging news from several of my friends here. Praise God!!!! I feel like we're one big family here.... although it's still not home, and we're all here because of our circumstances. Not here by choice and not for vacation, but we're making the best of it by clinging to, and leaning on, each other.

I always struggle with the first few days here with the homesickness, and the jetlag doesn't help. We've talked to our kids, granddad, and Janice at the house on SKYPE already and they are all doing great. I miss them. Janice, a friend from church, is taking care of my family this trip and I can't thank her enough! Today went by so very quickly. I pray the rest of the days here will too, but also that I can have some fun here as well. It's hot here today, but I'm so not complaining. We have a fan in our room which feels reminiscent of the "olden days", growing up in Florida without air-conditioning.

Tuesday, May 26, 2009 10:45 PM

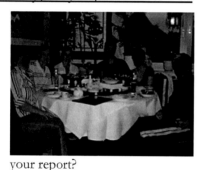

Questions and Answers

Question # 1 How's it going over there?

Question # 2 Is your room nice this time?

Question # 3 How's the weather?

Question #4 What has the doc had to say about your report?

Question # 5 Will you still get whole body hyperthermia this time?

Question # 6 If you do, will you get the low-dose kimo with it this time?

Question # 7 Do you know what the plan of action for the future is going to be?

These are the questions my sister-in-law, with the very active brain cells, has asked me to answer. They are very good questions so here are the answers so far.

#1 It's going very well here except we are still so tired, which is why these answers are so short.

#2 We are in one of the rooms that have Wi-Fi so at least Chuck and I can be on both laptops at the same time. The last trip, we had to take turns or bring the computer downstairs. We are sleeping in a bed that's a little smaller than a double. It's fine.

#3 The weather is hot but getting cooler as we speak and very windy today, delightful! There is no A/C here because they would only use it for a few weeks out of the year. We have a fan that we asked for and had a screen put on the window so we will be able to leave it open all night, yes! There are even bugs and mosquitoes in Germany! Last night with the window closed was quite hot, so by the time the nurse came in to check my vital signs this morning, I had very few PJs on.... whatever! After being naked for hyperthermia, it just doesn't matter. They've seen it all! It's much cooler tonight so it will be great to sleep with the window open.

#4 Dr. Herzog, of course, is excited about my report but has said I need to be aware there could still be microscopic cells present, which I was aware of, which is why I'm not changing anything about my healthy routine.

#5 and #6 Tomorrow I will be getting my Whole Body Hyperthermia(WBH) with the low-dose kimo as usual. It's important to finish the scheduled routine. Remember the comparison to finishing your antibiotics in order for them to be as effective as possible?

#7 Dr. Herzog has not had a chance to look at my MRI films yet. It's not like he was waiting at the front door for me and running immediately to his computer with them, unfortunately. Remember, I had to leave my first class status back at the plane, although they are great here. We asked him about the films today and he said he will talk to us as soon as he looks at them. He definitely understood our anxiousness in hearing from him so I'll have to finish that last question later!

I'm having my WBH tomorrow bright and early so say a prayer that they get my temp to exactly where God wants it and that I come through with no complications. I'll wake up at 6 am for the prepping and start the heating at around 7 am. Even though I've done this 3 times, I'm still nervous. At least I won't have to eat anything all day until dinner... yippee! I get so tired of Chuck telling me it's time to eat again, when I don't have any appetite. I know, I really don't need to lose any more weight. I'm at my perfect weight right now.

Tonight we went with 2 friends from Ocala, one from Colorado, and one from Australia to a Thai Restaurant (see picture). Delicious! We got 6 different dishes and shared everything. Yum! The waitress was very nice and brought out tiny glasses of plum wine for each of us. What the heck, it was very light and small. I had one.

When we got back to the clinic the nurse met me with two huge IVs, one with glucose and the other with saline, in preparation for tomorrow. I don't really remember getting these before. I'd rather just drink them. It would be a lot faster, but I know it's not the same. These won't finish until 2 am (remember my slow PICC line?) and I'll be getting up all night going to the bathroom! At least I get to sleep all day tomorrow! Everyone here knows when each of us is having WBH so they'll be asking Chuck how I'm doing, and then looking for me when I get out and about. It's so soothing to have such caring people here.

There's a new lady here from Greece who got here the same day we did. It's her first trip and she is very unhappy. I know how she feels. She misses home and doesn't want to be here. She says she's been crying a lot. I spoke with her tonight for a while and, with her permission, gave her 2 of my books to read. Both are small, easy to read faith and Christian books. I told her she could keep them the whole time we're here and that they really helped me get through some very rough places. She said she would read them.

Dr. Herzog stopped by our room around 10 pm to briefly go over tomorrow's WBH plan. This was comforting. Everything looks good! Wish me luck.

Wednesday, May 27, 2009 11:00 PM

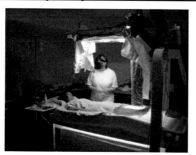

Highest Body Temperature Ever!

It's very late right now... 11:23 pm as we have just talked to the kids on SKYPE and I didn't even get up from my WBH until 8 pm tonight. They really did me up good!.... Exactly what I wanted. Dr. Herzog came to the treatment area himself and allowed my core body temp to get to 105.8 F for about half an hour and then 107.6 for a half hour.....

wow!!! And not one blister. My legs, and a few other areas, had red spots and marks as you can imagine, so the nurses were busy covering me with the icy cold silver nitrate cream and gauze and yes, white fishnet again, ooh la la!

Every time we met with Dr. Herzog we expressed our concern over the "measly" 104.3 F last time as he is the expert in Germany on "Extreme Heat Hyperthermia". I am so happy about the higher temp even though I felt much more tired afterwards. I remember them trying to wake me up but I was just so sleepy.

The only thing that hurts is the skin on my heels. Oops, that's my fault. I remember now that I gave myself a pedicure before coming back to Germany and really worked at removing all the cracked skin on my heels. Guess I overdid it. They even put sheepskin booties on my feet before starting, to protect the heels.

I struggled through dinner from the tiredness and lack of appetite, probably from reaching such a high temp today. It was worth it. I need to conserve some energy for a "spit bath" tonight (the gauze will be removed tomorrow).

I plan on venturing out briefly tomorrow to find some peony flower bushes. They are in bloom now. They have them here and I've never seen them on a bush before. Whole Foods in Florida sells them but are 14 dollars for 5 of them, so I've never purchased them. They are only available for about 2 weeks. My sister always talks about how beautiful they are in Chicago, and how wonderful they smell. I've always wanted to have some but they can't grow in Florida... too hot.

Thursday, May 28, 2009 9:30 PM

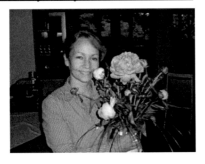

Peonies!

I'm having a really hard time shaking the tiredness today and slept quite a bit. We did manage to go out and find a peony bush with pink flowers! We also found a bouquet with a peony in the cafeteria (see picture)! There are a lot of other magnificent flowers in bloom here too. It's a little chilly and overcast today, but should warm up tomorrow.

I'm glad the day is almost over. I'm still holding on to about a gallon of fluid from yesterday's successful rampage. Tomorrow I'm sure I'll be a little lighter and less puffy. I don't like being this puffy, but still, it's worth it!

The sun comes up around 5 am and it stays light here until about 10 pm, so it's hard to get started on the evening routine early enough to get to bed on time. My stomach is not feeling quite right which is to be expected. There is medicine I can take for it.

We played Uno Spin with our friends from Texas so that was good for a few laughs. I lost the game, big time. I don't really have a whole lot to say about today. Just getting through it is all I'm after.

No word from Dr. Herzog about future treatments yet. My MRI pictures, from a major imaging center at home, are too small for him to see the details so he has to get them enlarged before he can tell us anything more.

Friday, May 29, 2009 10:30 PM

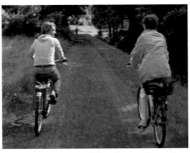

Bike Riding the German Countryside

The day started off slow with sleepiness. I had my local hyperthermia which made me get out of bed. I didn't feel like eating so Chuck got me something for later while I headed off to my appointment. After a while, Dr. Herzog came in and said my platelets were very low today and maybe my body is getting tired of getting kimo.... duh! I agree! I asked if I got more this time than last and he said "No, it's the exact same amount each time". Maybe it was the higher temp then that caused more tiredness and puffiness this time, we're thinking. He said exercise will help improve my platelets.... guess I'll have to get outside and do something instead of sleeping all day, which is what I'd rather do.

For lunch we had salmon, yucky smell, but then actually quite tasty and I ate quite a bit. The chef was cooking it fresh on the griddle. At lunch our French lady friend, Michaelina, suggested we go bike riding with her. After a long nap, I decided that would be energizing and fun, so we headed to the bike shop for rental bikes.

To sum it up, she had us pedaling all over town, through wheat and corn fields, through woods and up and down big hills (see picture). Our bikes also had those cute little ring ring bells on the handlebars. I thought I was in decent shape but I guess kimo and a 107 degree temp takes a toll on a person. At least, I was the only one who didn't actually fall off their bike............ Yes, Chuck was with us too. He was showing off when he fell off and Michaelina was not watching where she was going when she headed off into a ditch. Fortunately, the grass was soft and no one got hurt! I suppose they just thought I needed a good laugh, and it worked!

We rode for over an hour and stopped to smell all kinds of flowers I had never seen before. There were lots of Peonies... gorgeous... in all different colors. It was quite the workout! Now isn't this exactly what the doctor ordered?

Tonight, dinner was actually not bad with tortellinis and alfredo sauce. Then we watched one of my favorite movies, Get Smart. I invited the lady from Greece, and her husband, to watch with us. She didn't stay for the whole thing, although I'm not sure why, but her husband stayed. At least she knows I thought of her. She seems down and I totally understand that.

We are still waiting for a decision from Dr. Herzog as far as "what's next" for me. Please pray for divine guidance for him regarding my care.

Saturday, May 30, 2009 10:45 PM

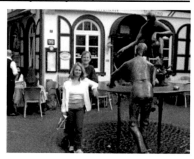

A Day in Giessen

I'm really missing home as there is a lot going on there. Tyler leaves for camp on Sunday, and Morgan is going to see a movie with some friends AND a guy! First date, sort of, and I'm here! Some days I just have to go minute by minute. At least today was sunny and delightful and we got out and enjoyed the warmth and beauty.

We went to the city of Giessen where there were many wonderful shops. There were lots of people out enjoying the area. It's amazing how many locals ride their bikes everywhere. We got there at 1 pm and I thought we would be picked up around 3 or 4 but the driver said he couldn't come back until 6.... hmmm. That's a long time to be stuck somewhere. I was concerned I would get overly tired,

We went with another couple from Texas and a man from Scotland. We found a sandwich shop like Panera's, at home, and really took our time eating. I ate this huge sandwich. We splurged and got a fresh strawberry dessert "thing" which was marvelous. The desserts here are not loaded with sugar, by the way, like they are in the U.S. Getting outside to some fresh air and sunshine really improves my appetite and energy... it's amazing!

We didn't buy very much. It was just nice to be out and about. We stopped for some drinks as my legs were getting very tired which made my stomach not feel too good. I had a "bitter lemon" drink which is a lightly sweetened refreshing "bitter" lemonade. It really hit the spot for me.

On the way back we were suddenly at a McDonald's. How did that happen? We're in Germany, at McDonald's! I figured I might as well eat now and get it over with, and splurge again. It did smell good in there. I had a big sized chicken wrap, which I don't think they have at home. It was full-sized with lettuce and tomato and was oh, so yummy. I even had 3 French fries!

I'm already planning on what we're going to do tomorrow away from the klinik. I think we might go bike riding again and try to find the airfield and maybe where that glider comes from. The masseuse Jeanine slid a note under the door today letting me know there was an airfield on the way to Nidda just over the hill. We were talking about it yesterday during my massage. That was so sweet of her. She said she was going to try to find info on the internet and she did! Now for the next question. How much is it to glide through the air without an engine? MasterCard and priceless? I don't think so.

My platelets were a little higher today... yay. From 61,000 to 73,000. It means they are on their way up. They'll be checked again on Monday.

I gave the lady from Greece several hugs this evening as she will be leaving for home early in the morning. She is not able to stay for treatment at this time due to inflammation of the vein in her thigh. She plans on coming back next month though.

Several of you have asked me to let you know of any specific prayer needs I have. Well, I do. Perseverance, peace, joy and of course thankfulness for continued healing. Even though it sounds like I'm having a ball here, this is really wearing on me, yet I want to do what I need to do, to get well. Thank you all for continuing to support me by conversing with us through this wonderful invention, the internet!

Sunday, May 31, 2009 9:45 PM

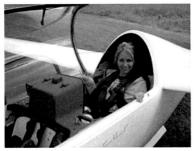

Gliding through the Air!

We did it!!!!!!!!!!!! We rode in the glider plane.... woohoo!!!!!!! It was awesome! More exciting than any ride or roller coaster, ever! We rented bikes and headed out to find the airfield. We made a few wrong turns and had lots of steep hills to cover but with the help of some locals, we found it.

One problem, we entered by way of the landing field! Here come two bikers right where the planes land. The people were a little upset, asking if we read the signs. In my sweetest voice I said I'm sorry, we can't read German. There were several men, some kids, a mom, and two teenage boys there. I felt like we were intruding on a family outing.

It was hard to start a conversation but I wanted to ride. I started asking about the gliders and how fascinated we've been with seeing them overhead for months. Then they started asking about why we were here for months. We said "medical reasons" and left it at that.

I asked if they give rides and if so how much are they. The older man said, Yes we do, it's 15 euros for 10 minutes of air time unless you want the newer big glider then it's 20 for 10 minutes. At that time the big glider landed and all of them went to push it over to where we were standing. Chuck had only brought 30 euros. The pilot of the newer plane came over and said he spoke a little English. Turns out he works for IBM and is very fluent! The men spoke in German for a few seconds and then the pilot said I'll give you both a ride for 30, a discount. I was ecstatic and we were so appreciative.

What an amazing person he was. He explained everything in detail that he was doing and why. He first had me put on the parachute.... what????? He said it was my cushion to lean against. My next question was, where is the rip cord? I said I wouldn't touch it unless I was free falling. Then I got in and he started strapping me in. I made sure I knew how to unstrap each of those. He closed the clear lid and I had to fight a little bit of claustrophobia. There was a tiny little vent in the window which I quickly opened for fresh air. It helped.

The way they get the glider up into the sky is by a huge wench (made by GM, he added). It was on the back of a truck way over on the other side of the hill at least a half mile away. Suddenly we took off fast, kind of like The Hulk ride at Universal but not as bad. In 3 seconds we were climbing up at about a 60 degree angle, very fast... awesome. He said we will get up to 180 km/hr in those 3 seconds.

Looking down, I couldn't believe how far up we were, so quickly. I heard a loud "clunk" which scared me. I thought a wing fell off! He quickly said it's ok, it's just the winch line dropping off. We circled and he explained how they use the thermal drafts to rise higher and higher, and how you can feel them when you hit one, a little lifting on one of the wings. When you turn into it, you rise higher. He said that's how the birds do it too and they both often end up flying around in the same patterns.

We circled a lot, big circles, to get very high. I don't even know how high. I was just in awe. Then he asked me if I wanted to do 2 "G's" in order to experience zero gravity for a few seconds. And do that twice. I thought for a few seconds and said a resounding "yes!"

What a wild ride! Dive bombing for about 3 seconds, then the 2 G's would occur as we pulled straight up out of it... super, heavy pressure on my whole body, then back down to have the zero gravity where you feel a slight lifting from your seat, only as much as the straps would allow... just a few seconds, unfortunately. I actually started crying a little I was so excited. I quickly let him know I was just emotional because it was so awesome.

We circled a little bit more. I even saw the klinik from up there. Before long, it was landing time. I'm usually so scared landing on a commercial flight but this was nothing. A little bumpiness as we passed closely over the trees, which he explained causes some drafts, and then some slight bumps as we landed on the hard grassy landing strip before coming to a gradual easy stop.

It was so awesome actually being able see where we were going, unlike on the big planes. That made a huge difference in making it not scary. He was so good at explaining everything that we were doing, and why, and the different sounds and how it all works and what we were doing next and how I would feel. All that in 10 minutes???? I don't think so! More like 20 or more. I think he was having fun showing off his glider skills for me. Then it was Chuck's turn! I'll explain his trip now.... "Ditto"!.... except I don't THINK he cried!

When we left we went a different way back that was NOT on the landing field! If anyone ever gets the chance to do this, DO IT. It's not near as wild as a rollercoaster ride but somehow, so much more incredible. And we didn't have to do those "G's" and dips but "Yes" just came out of my mouth all by itself.

Oh yeah, I had infusions and a nice un-eventful visit from the Dr.

Monday, June 1, 2009 11:15 PM

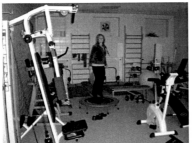

Laughter, Truly Great Medicine

Obviously today was not as exciting as yesterday. I can't believe how many people don't want to go in the glider plane. What is wrong with them?????? There are 3 men here at the klinik that would be willing... that's it!

Dr. Herzog was thrilled that we went. He likes to fly and ride bikes. He headed out today in all his bicycle gear, bright colors and all. I better be careful or he just might have me returning if he thinks I'm having so much fun....

Today I slept as long as possible and even planned on a nap. The pillows here are like huge square flat lumpy things. I haven't been sleeping very well and dream of my own pillow when I'm trying to get comfortable. I ended up reading in bed today instead of napping, which was fine, but tomorrow morning and each morning after this my local hyperthermias will be getting me up around 8 am or earlier.... ughhh. But closer and closer to Friday! Only 3 more days left.

I decided my muscles needed a boost so we went to exercise for 10 minutes (see picture) and ended up doing yoga for another 35 minutes. It felt great! I was exhausted, in a really good way. There were no workers in the massage area since it's technically a holiday similar to our Memorial Day so...... I treated Chuck to a very much needed massage on a real "massage table". Of course, he said I was better than the masseuse. I tried to speak in a German accent to make it authentic but I don't think he bought it.

Tonight we ordered pizza (lightening up a little on my diet), and I also got a salad. I even had a small cup of coke. I don't normally even drink soda but, wow was it good! It's nice to have a change of food, occasionally, from the klinik. The main course here tonight was pancakes stuffed with blueberry filling.... although it does sound good, but not for dinner, you silly people. Again, lunch is the main meal here. Dinner is usually very light.

Tonight we played Uno Spin with our favorite friends from Texas again. When we all get together like that I sure get to laughing really hard just at the silliest little things that turn into big things. I tell you, hard laughing sure makes a not-so-good-feeling stomach feel a lot better.

Here's an example of the silliness. Antje, the nurse, came walking in with a patient's little black 11 month old baby. The baby was wearing cute PJs with strawberries on them. Our friend Rodney told Antje to "shake her up and down just a little", which she did, and the baby liked. Then Rodney said, "Now you have a chocolate-strawberry shake!" Antje actually "got it" pretty quickly... did you???? The whole table burst into laughter!

My platelets are on the rise, 115,000 today. White and red blood cells are up too.... excellent. They were down just a little this time.

Tuesday, June 2, 2009 10:15 PM

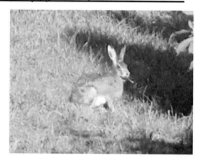

Dr. Herzog says, "Complete Remission"!

I am super tired tonight, which is good. You're supposed to be tired at night. I've tried to nap today but have just been too busy, which is also good. It made the day go by faster. To bed at 1 am and up at 7 just doesn't work well. Now that I have a nice pillow (asked for a softer one from the house keeper), there's no time to sleep! Up again tomorrow morning at 7 for my other big day. I'll be getting one of the two kimo's along with my local hyperthermia treatment at 9 am so I'll need to start the pre-kimo IV at around 7:30. Another early morning.

I feel a little more upbeat today since we only have 2 more full days then we go home! I cried for Dr. Herzog this morning. It wasn't hard. He asked me how I was and that's all it took. I told him I was so homesick and didn't want to come back. He said, "but you're having so much fun here with biking and plane gliding".... yes, but still, I'm homesick. I told him yesterday that I don't want kimo anymore.... we all know that's obvious. I told him today that my hair is beginning to fall out. It's everywhere, in the shower, on the floor, in bed, I even found one in Chuck's food......my ponytail is thinner. It seems my hair is about one-third less thick than usual. I may have exaggerated just a little to make a statement to let him know that I think my body is done with this stuff..

But.......... today in my room he was with my chart explaining my situation to a new doctor and I heard him say "now in complete remission". He was talking about me! Although I don't care for the word "remission"........ I think "cured" would be better to hear...... it's still a great word to hear from your oncologist! With that, I started crying again but just for emotional reasons. I still have it in my head that he may want me to come back soon and that in its self can make me cry.

After he left the room I finally realized what he had said and started crying again because I had not heard him say that about me before... the "remission" part. He is so calm natured but you would think he would grab my shoulders and scream it to me in excitement! Again, in between crying, he said he was going for a total cure so that I would be able to forget about all this down the road. That's what I'm going for but I will never forget! All this has done so much to, and for, me.

We had lunch with my Texas friend Becky and her husband, and she said she cried the whole time he was in her room too. She's only 2 doors down from me. The doctors were probably wondering what was going on today. The new doctor is probably thinking we're always like that here. We went out for dinner again with Becky and her husband, and Vera from Munich, who arrived today. She's always a pleasure to spend time with and always has new information to share about cancer treatments. She's the "energizer bunny" of talking about new and existing treatments in Germany and elsewhere. She brings interesting information to Dr. Herzog every time she comes here.... about once a month, and he actually listens to her! I like hearing her opinion on things and her fascinating stories. She's very bright and has lived quite an adventurous life!

Wow, it's 10 pm, it's just about dark, but the birds are still going strong. They must be exhausted too!!!!! They'll be waking up in only 7 hours. Earlier, when we looked out our window there was a huge rabbit "walloping" across the lawn. He was so big he did not even hop. At first I thought it was a gazelle with huge ears.... odd for me to think a gazelle is on the lawn in Germany, but that's what it looked like. I named him Peter and he was adorable. See the cute picture!

Wednesday, June 3, 2009 11:30 PM

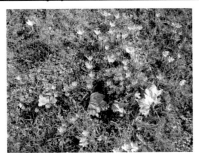

Harness His Power!

We have been "socializing" for hours and it's been a very pleasant day in spite of receiving "kimo" this morning during my local hyperthermia. Of course I had to insist they start my infusions very early as my IV line runs so slowly. They said no, I said yes, and explained again why, I made my case calmly and my pre-kimo was running within 20 minutes.... yessss! Everything worked out perfectly! Chuck even brought me a nice breakfast since I'm not allowed to leave the area with "kimo paraphernalia". I was in an easy chair with a blanket over my lap. I felt like I was on first class again with Chuck and one of my favorite nurses as my flight attendants.....(smile).

Please everyone pray hard tonight for divine guidance from the Holy Spirit directly to Dr. Herzog's mind! He will let us know tomorrow what he decides is the best ongoing treatment plan for me.... sigh.

Today, I had a very small but very meaningful answer to a prayer. As you know I've been trying to take a nap for a few days. I finally laid down in bed at 2:15 pm. My eyes were wide open and I could think of all these things I'd rather be doing. My brain just wouldn't stop. I couldn't relax at all even though I knew my body needed the rest. I decided to say a quick one sentence prayer for a very nice, specifically a "deep" sleep. I can't believe I didn't even get to "amen" and suddenly my body and jaw felt as if I were in a paralyzed state. I could not move and for the first time since being here, was ever so comfortable. There were NO more thoughts whatsoever.......

Next thing I knew, my eyes were open and the light in the room had changed. I looked at my watch and it had been 2 and a half hours. I was even in the exact same position, my hands and everything! Even the pant leg of Chuck's pajamas was still over my eyes where I had placed it to block the light. It was a sleep that felt like the result of getting IV sedation or something, a really "deep" sleep that goes by in a snap (No, men, this will not work on your wife when you think she's talking too much. I know that God thinks whatever your wife has to say is very important!). I realized as soon as I awoke that I have not slept like that...... since I can remember. And I felt the assurance of God's continual presence with me and realized how much more would He be with me during the bigger times.

Things like this are starting to happen to me. Little answers to little prayers. Things that tell me He is here, always, such as the beauty and fun we keep stumbling upon, and the people that make me laugh here every day. I feel He knew I needed all that to get through my time here. I am enjoying "harnessing the power" that is available to each of us that I have never really experienced before. I've heard of these things happening for other people but I can't honestly say they have happened for me on a regular basis in my life, until now. There is a verse about "being still" so God can speak with us. Our lives are so very busy. During my treatments I am alone and "still". About 1 to 2 hours each day of nothing else to do but lay there with my book, staring. I'm actually liking that time now, whereas before, Chuck would have to stay with me in order for me to be ok and get through it.

The book I'm studying is by Joyce Meyer "Battlefield of the Mind". She and I are so much alike. She has verses and then explains in more detail about each verse and how they relate to life. For the last 2 days I have been repeating Isaiah 30:18. It has had a significance for me. Here is how she writes it. "And therefore, the Lord waits (expecting, looking, and longing) to be gracious to you, and therefore He lifts Himself up, that He may have mercy on you and show loving-kindness to you. For the Lord is a God of justice. Blessed (happy, fortunate, to be envied) are all those who (earnestly) wait for Him (His victory, His favor, His love, His peace, His joy, and His matchless, unbroken companionship)!"

I would say He has been very gracious, showing mercy, and loving kindness to us!!!

<u>Thursday, June 4, 2009 8:30 PM</u>

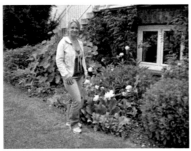

No More Kimo!

Coming home tomorrow!!! Pictured are the flowers we viewed from our room each day, roses and peonies in front of a pretty little quaint home, and……….ok, here's what Dr. Herzog said at our meeting today…..I'm in Complete Remission and I do not have to return next month! And no more kimo! He does want me to come back for a follow-up in 3 or 4 months for another whole body hyperthermia without kimo. I'm thinking that trip will only be a week, or less.

Also, based on clinical studies, he does not suggest any surgery since everything is gone. However he does want me to speak to a radiation oncologist about radiating the breast. That is his area of concern, not the lymph nodes. I was so dreading that he might want me one more time next month.

So now…… I'm thinking about having my PICC line removed as soon as I get home unless I can think of a reason to keep it. I'll have to think about that. I can't wait to swim and be able to shower like a normal person, especially with the warm weather we are into now.

Dr. Herzog wants me to finish my Thymus injections, of which I have 3 weeks left, and then start on Iscador M injections (Mistletoe from the apple tree). This means I am on a maintenance plan! The meds were just delivered from the pharmacy. The instructions for the dosaging are very confusing, so I just spoke with Dr. Herzog again and got it all straightened out. It's not an exact science like conventional medicine.

Thank you for all the prayers! This is what I wanted Dr. Herzog to tell me, for the most part. Now, I need guidance for what is next. Chuck and I celebrated by going for a walk and taking pictures of flowers. I've said my goodbyes to all the nurses, massage therapists, patients and everyone else. Everyone is so encouraged with my news. I'm still "on guard" as we still have a lot of homework to do to keep my health going in the right direction.

I must go now to help Chuck pack. I have to wake up at 5 am to complete my 5 infusions before heading out the door at 7:45 am. I don't think I'll be able to sleep very well.... I'm too excited!

Again, thank you ALL for the prayers and wonderful words of encouragement you have given me and the little things you say that make me laugh and sometimes cry, with joy! All of your words have meant so much to both Chuck and me.

Friday, June 5, 2009 8:00 PM

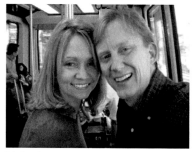

Back Home and Loving it!

Just a quick note that we made it home safe and sound. The flights were quite pleasant and I'm looking forward to my own bed tonight. Hopefully soon!

Additionally, I will be taking Morgan and Evan to week-long away camp on Sunday and bringing Tyler home. I can't wait to see him also! With driving all day on Sunday, I won't be able to see all of my "church family" until next week. I'm jumping right into things and loving every minute of it!

Wednesday, October 28, 2009 9:30 PM

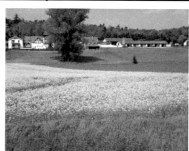

Hormonal Balance

Great news again! I had another MRI on Friday Oct. 23rd and just found out that it's totally normal, just like my last one 4 and a half months ago. It was quite stressful waiting for these results. I am so relieved and I praise God for all He is providing for my healing.

Upon my return from Germany last time, I had my hormones tested by way of "saliva" (yes, that's spit I'm referring to). Testing the saliva rather than the blood shows a more accurate level of the hormones "available" for use by the body. This testing showed my progesterone to be VERY low, causing an "estrogen-dominant" effect in my body. Dr. Herzog said he feels this dominance was a huge factor in causing the cancer in the first place. Since the type of cancer cells found in my body had both estrogen and progesterone receptors on the cells, the high levels of bad estrogens coupled with the low levels of progesterone in my body, spurred the cancer's growth. These levels can be thrown out of balance due to lifestyle factors, including diet and stress, "been there, done that!"

The saliva testing was done here at home, very inexpensively I might add, through a Compounding Pharmacist. I've been using the bio-identical progesterone and just had another saliva test done which shows my progesterone level is on the rise. However, an even higher level is needed to provide better protection against the estrogens causing another cancer issue. The progesterone I use is an over-the-counter, measured amount of cream, applied 20 days a month to the skin, super easy for such huge results! This was what was recommended to me by the Compounding Pharmacist who specializes in women's hormonal imbalances. There is also reference material on my website about progesterone and estrogen issues in dealing with breast cancer.

In addition, one thing Dr. Herzog wanted me to consider, which we have certainly felt strongly against, is radiation to the breast where the primary site WAS, but not the axilla where the affected lymph nodes were. He said radiation to the under-arm area causes a great deal of long-term effects due to the vast amount of nerve tissue located there. He also stated that the primary site could be the one more likely to cause a re-occurrence, not so much with the lymph nodes. I've seen firsthand the damage radiation treatment can cause and the wrecked immune system that follows. We've researched this aspect of treatment and have decided to forego it for now. It is something we have discovered, through researching, that can permanently damage the immune system even more so than kimo. We feel the immune system will play a key role in preventing cancer from re-occurring.

We will be heading back to Germany again with my "clear" MRI results to show Dr. Herzog on November 3rd through the 8th for another Whole Body Hyperthermia session with some high-dose IV vitamin C (without kimo), daily local hyperthermia sessions and some detox and immune boosting IVs before heading back home......."kick it while it's down" kind of thing.

Fifth Trip To Germany

Wednesday, November 4, 2009 10:00 PM

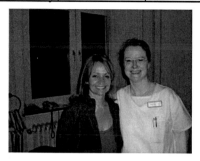

Feeling at Home in Germany

Once again, back in Germany. On the way from the airport, even though it was gloomy, aka cold and cloudy, there were some gorgeous yellow and orange trees and a brightly colored full rainbow, of which we could see both ends touching the ground. The ground was actually glowing where the rainbow's ends touched it.

As soon as we arrived I knew just what to do, run around getting my schedule filled with local hyperthermia appointments, giving hugs to nurses (see picture – me and Antje), the cafeteria ladies, my favorite housekeeper, etc. Of course, the first one I called to schedule was the masseuse.

Traveling across 6 times zones is exhausting so next, it was naptime for an hour, my massage, then nap for an hour, then local hyperthermia, then nap for 2 hours, then dinner at the Italian restaurant across the street with some friends. Still not caught up on sleep yet, but at least the plane trip was very uneventful.....a perfect word to describe both plane flights AND anything medical……..""uneventful""!

There are several patients (friends now) here that we know from before so will have to get busy visiting since we have a lot of catching up to do with them and only a few days to do it. Friday is my whole body hyperthermia which makes that day a "wash" as far as socializing. I'll be in "la la land", then only capable of smiling and nodding.

Ouch... I just got my IV started..... two sticks.... where are my favorite IV nurses???? I'm receiving B vitamins and vitamin C 7.5 grams, for starters. Now I get to walk around with this "Lock", or IV plug, in my arm. Good thing I took a nice shower earlier since now I'll have to hang my arm out of the shower or wrap it up to keep it dry.

It's bedtime for these bunnies (Chuck and me) so "signing off".

Thursday, November 5, 2009 11:00 PM

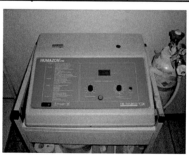

Lesson – Ozone Therapy and Intravenous Vitamin C

Today I had a new procedure, new for me that is. Instead of my usual injection of ozone in the hip area, they did something different where they drained my blood from my arm into a glass bottle like when you donate blood but only about half a cup. Then the nurse injected 45 units of "ozone" air into the bottle and swirled the bottle to mix the ozone into the blood. My usual injection in the hip is only 15 units of ozone (pictured is the ozone machine with the tank of ozone next to it on the right). The bottle was then raised high allowing the blood to infuse back into my arm. It was all done very quickly in about 15 minutes with the needle remaining in my arm and connected by the tubing to the bottle the entire time……..very strange, but supposedly more effective at getting more ozone into me.

A different doctor was here today and ordered ozone this way, so I gave it a try. I'm here for such a short time that I'm only getting my ozone injection once anyway. I'm so done with needles today. I've had 4 since last night. Each time seems to hurt more.

I've forgotten exactly what ozone therapy does since I read about it months ago, so I looked it up and found this. I'm glad I went for the bigger dose!

According to Frank Shallenberger, MD, author of The Principles and Applications of Ozone Therapy, "bio-oxidative therapies" (aka, ozone therapy) affect the human body in the following ways:

- They stimulate the production of white blood cells, which are necessary to fight infection.
- Ozone and hydrogen peroxide are virucidal (virus-killing).
- They increase oxygen and hemoglobin disassociation, thus increasing the delivery of oxygen from the blood to the cells.
- Ozone and hydrogen peroxide are anti-neoplastic, which means that they inhibit the growth of new tissues such as tumors.
- They oxidize and degrade petrochemicals.
- They increase red blood cell membrane flexibility and effectiveness.
- Bio-oxidative therapies increase the production of interferon and Tumor Necrosis Factor, which the body uses to fight infections and cancers.
- They increase the efficiency of the anti-oxidant enzyme system, which scavenges excess free radicals in the body.
- They accelerate the citric acid cycle, which is the main cycle for the liberation of energy from sugars. This then stimulates basic metabolism.
- Bio-oxidative therapies increase tissue oxygenation, thus bringing about patient improvement.

I wish I could have that machine at home!

Today was like yesterday, sleepy and rainy. I did manage to make it to the gym for some mini-trampoline jumping and a little yoga. I've been feeling stiff since the plane ride. I'm doing ok with the food here since there's no kimo involved this trip. Tomorrow I make my way to the hyperthermia room downstairs for the heating session, for which I've travelled from afar.

Interesting, this time since I won't be getting any kimo, they will be infusing an even higher dose of vitamin C than usual, 30 grams, yes that's an infusion of the equivalent of thirty, 1000mg tablets. This is done at my peak temperature in the place of kimo. I have received 25 grams before at my alternative doctor's office with no side effects. Again, I looked up exactly how high dose vitamin C works and found some interesting reading at www.orthomolecular.org/library/ivccancerpt.shtml. It explains how intravenous vitamin C actually gets into the cancer cells and turns into "hydrogen peroxide", which is lethal to the cancer cells. But this can only be accomplished through the IV route, not with oral tablets. At the same time there is no damage to healthy cells. In fact it's given by integrative physicians at home to help combat colds, flu, and other ailments.

At this time, Chuck and I are reading a book I just bought and I can't wait to finish it. He keeps telling me the things he's reading and it's fantastic what the doctors in the book are accomplishing. It's Suzanne Somers latest called "Knockout". It is interviews with alternative cancer treatment doctors in the U.S. who have been curing people of all different types of cancers. It's great information for anyone wanting to stay in the U.S. for treatments, as well as a chapter on suggestions for supportive therapies for those who choose regular, conventional treatments.

Say a prayer for me tomorrow, 11 am my time, 5 am your time. So set your alarm clocks....just kidding. But I do want the prayers anyway no matter what time it is.

Friday, November 6, 2009 10:00 PM

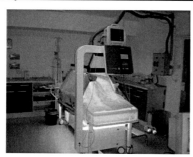

Hyperthermia Chamber/Vitamin C instead of Chemo

I slept so much today that Chuck had to tell me how I did for my WBH and the rest of the day. I slept on and off since I finished my WBH treatment. Everything went great! I was heated up to 40.9 C or 105.62 F. Perfect, that's right where we wanted to be! (pictured is me all tucked in, monitors in place, and ready for the session).

I received my high dose of IV vitamin C as planned, and as usual I did get some red blotches on my legs, but those will be gone by tomorrow. My left toe, next to the big toe, got burned some again. It happens to that spot every time....very strange. But like the flight over here, it seems my WBH was "uneventful". Outstanding!

Tomorrow we hope to get out and do some sightseeing or shopping. After spending the whole day inside today, we will need some fresh air and exercise.

Saturday, November 7, 2009 9:00 PM

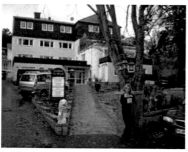

Gearing Up To Come Home

I had to get stuck again today. My IV line just quit working. I'm hoping this IV will last one more time for tomorrow morning. I don't like needles and I'm getting so tired of them. Gotta do what ya gotta do though!

It's time to start packing to come home already! Still waiting for the doctor to come visit me and tell us what's next. I had my ultrasound today and all was normal as I expected but still nerve wracking. My blood work came back normal as well, also as I expected. Today I've been recovering from feeling like a tired blimp. Doing better now but I guess even without kimo I retain a lot of fluid. Chuck and I were wondering if it was the heat or kimo that causes the swelling after each WBH. It's the heat! This makes sense because during the Florida summers, my rings feel tighter. Fortunately, all the wrinkles were gone from my face. Unfortunately, I could barely open my eyes and my hands kept falling asleep. Getting outside and walking always helps. I'm actually happy to have those little wrinkles back.

We managed to take a long walk outside in the park behind the klinik. There were lots of brightly colored trees but again it was very wet and chilly, about 45 degrees F. You'd think with all that vitamin C I'd be full of energy but no, I think the cold, wet, cloudy weather is stronger than any vitamin. It'll be great to get home where it's not so humid and freezing. Imagine, a place more humid than Florida, that would be here!

We'll be leaving here around 7 am and flying out at 9:45 am, arriving in Orlando around 5:27 pm, of course after taking off the 6 hour time difference. I love landing in Orlando. It's so comforting to be home again. Here's to another boring flight home! Remember, in this case, boring and uneventful is extraordinary!

Saturday, November 14, 2009 3:00 PM

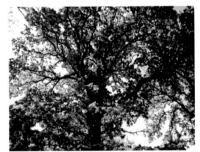

Iscador Lesson (Immune Stimulator)

Upon arriving home, I immediately jumped back into life. Making such a short trip definitely made the transition to the time back home much easier. I'm back to everything healthy, with an occasional piece of candy or chocolate here and there, back to my exercising and enjoying the nice warm weather. The paybacks for all this healthy eating are great.... for one thing, my favorite jeans ALWAYS fit and I have lots of energy without caffeine.

We met with Dr. Herzog the night before we left and he said everything was perfectly normal. No signs of any problems. However, we need to keep our guard up by continuing the healthy lifestyle and get an MRI periodically. I will have an MRI in a few months, move to every 6 months for the next year, and then probably go to yearly tests. This will be ordered by my integrative physician at home.

Dr. Herzog wants me to continue taking Iscador. Iscador is an immune stimulator, processed from mistletoe (yes, the kind you see growing high in trees and used for nabbing kisses!) Dr. Herzog has prescribed Iscador M which comes from the mistletoe that grows on the apple tree. Mistletoe has a slightly different composition depending on the tree it's attached to. Different types are prescribed depending on the type of cancer being treated. This means mistletoe is not just a parasite on a tree, but a healing medicine.

The dosing method is confusing since it's not an exact science. The way each person's dose is calculated is this; the initial very small dose is increased over a period of several weeks until a small local 1 inch reaction occurs. The correct dose for that person is then the previous dose that did not cause the reaction. For example, the first month I took

0.5 mg twice a week, then moved to 0.7 mg twice a week. Each time I would try the next higher dose, I would get a reaction (meaning an area of redness at least 1 inch in diameter at the injection site). The doctor said that the 0.7 mg dose should work just fine. That's the dose I will stay on indefinitely. We brought home a lot of Iscador from the German pharmacy before we left since you can't get it from here. Booooo!

The doctor also wants to see me in 6 months or so for another follow up with whole body and local hyperthermia's. Chuck and I are pretty sure he will always suggest we come back for a follow-up because if he didn't, and something happened….Dr. Herzog wants to be sure I stay safe, so I know it will ultimately be up to Chuck and me when we decide I don't need to return. We hope to go two more times, one this coming year and one the next.

Chuck and I want to, again, thank everyone so much for all the help and support provided for us. Without it, we just don't know how we could've made it through this scary year as we depended on so much help for our family as well as the emotional support and prayers.

Cancer Is a Lifestyle Issue

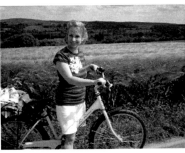

Since cancer is a lifestyle issue, I plan on doing what I need to do in order to keep it a "thing of the past". It was my "wake-up call" that I lived to tell about!

Since my trips to Germany I've been following a regimen of supplements, exercise, yoga, stress reducing techniques, and power napping instead of "pushing through" with ANOTHER cup of coffee like I used to do. I'm also juicing almost every day, eating as many fruits and veggies as I can (which is getting easier), and using simple bio-identical progesterone.

I continue to detox on a daily basis through drinking lemon water, green powdered supplementing, heavy dooty fiber drinks (sorry, couldn't resist that) different teas (yum), such as chamomile, green tea, rooiboos, Pau' d arco, etc. A lot of the stuff I do is easy, it just requires a change of lifestyle which takes time and organization. More info about my different regimens, teas, and detoxing is also on my website, www.AHealthyApproach.com.

All of this sounds like a lot of work, and it was at first, but now it's just becoming a part of my lifestyle that I've grown accustomed to. I actually feel better physically and mentally than I ever have in my life at any age, and without any caffeine, alcohol, or red meat. So far it has been well worth the effort.

Things are finally coming together now. I have a plan for good health, my treatments have wound down, and I feel so amazing, physically and mentally. Putting all this "in black and white" actually causes me to feel somewhat shaky and teary eyed with excitement.

Don't misunderstand me, I do not feel I am totally out of the "scary woods" I was in, and I don't have my "head in the sand". We pray a lot for guidance and continue to research and read about different aspects of treatments with a very open mind. How else would I have wound up in Germany for cancer treatments without a COMPLETELY OPEN MIND?

Fast forward to 2014.
<u>Where am I now, almost 6 years later?</u>...........

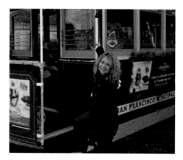

Still cancer free and a lot wiser for it..........dare I say, my life is so much better now than before? I do have a deeper appreciation for the meaning and value of life and the little things that make each day awesome.

Looking back on those scary days, I am still so thankful for the friends I made at the clinic. We all leaned on each other and found such comfort in knowing we weren't there alone, along with the laughter we all shared. One couple in particular still stands out in my memory.

That couple is Becky and Rodney from Texas. They rode with us in the van from the airport to the clinic. It was both of our first trips to Germany! Come to find out, we were even on the same plane from the states! We got to know one another in the van as "scared newbies" coming to Germany for cancer treatment.

We developed a special bond right from the start as we all entered the clinic together, figuring out what to do and where to go first. Becky ended up becoming my best friend there and a lifesaver during that, and subsequent trips. Her natural ability to do and say "stupid" things and then laugh at herself is what had us all in hysterics many times each and every day! Her husband said she was like that all the time! It went both ways. I feel that I also helped her through some times when she felt scared. I still chuckle and feel good when I think about her......and then I thank God for her.

We have not kept in contact over the years, which is ok. I feel that God places people in our lives as we need them, and she was one of those special "God placed" souls when He knew I needed that laughter. In turn, I felt I was a support person for her as well.

I'm happy to say that Pastor Tom made a full recovery from the heart attack suffered during our first trip to the clinic. He changed his diet, even though he doesn't like to admit this, and is still the usual fantastic fun-loving preacher who continues to make church both "fun and refreshing"! Praise the Lord! He and his lovely wife Carol have continued to be two of our closest friends.

Life changing situations cause us to change our priorities. Sometimes a friend will remind me of how I left my Christmas tree up, and decorated, the entire year I was having my treatments. Yes, that's right, I did! I forget about that sometimes. My house always had to be perfect or I wore myself out trying to make it that way! During that year, I realized that taking down the tree was not a priority at that time. My health, my family and the people in my life were the only things that mattered. Sometimes life forces you to put things on the "back burner". Then you realize what you thought was important means ABSOLUTELY NOTHING in the grand scheme of things.

For example, little things used to cause me a lot of stress. I would allow things to throw off my whole demeanor and I could feel my anxiety building........a messy house, ruined clothing from a pen going through the laundry, a child's room filled with chaos as if a tornado struck, making dinner and the sink is overflowing with dishes, or having to change plans for the day because of car problems. I thought this was "who I was" and that I couldn't change it. I learned I was wrong about that.

I've learned to take a step back, think, and purposely try to deal with those irritations in a more logical and calm manner. This is better for my health and the health of my family. People are more important than "things", ALWAYS. These things are still an inconvenience and I do become annoyed at times. My kids still have to clean their rooms and do the dishes, but I try to make my reaction more purposeful than "flying off the handle".

Another priority is myself. Since my "wake-up call" and my time in Germany, I make time for taking care of myself, physically and mentally, just like at the clinic. I allow my mistakes to be made without being overly critical of myself. I've learned my perfectionism can be my enemy if I let it. While I still struggle at times to go easy on myself, I tell myself, tomorrow is another day, another opportunity to do it better. And it's going to be a great day!

Tschuss! pronounced "choos", which is "bye" in German.

ABOUT THE AUTHOR

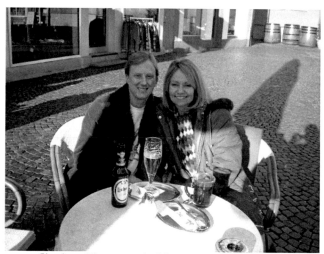

Chuck and Laura in the Plaza at the center of Nidda

Laura Jackson has been a Registered Nurse since 1983 and works as a healthcare educator for a major hospital system in central Florida. She is married and has three children.

After winning her battle against stage 3 breast cancer in 2009, she started AHealthyApproach.com. A website that is dedicated to providing information on natural, common sense approaches to improving one's current health condition as well as suggestions to making your health a priority. As most mothers, she always took better care of those around her than herself. However, after the harrowing ordeal with cancer, she now takes the time needed and has priorities in place to do the important things in life as well as instilling healthier habits in her 3 children, so that they, hopefully, won't fall into the trap of thinking, "all my friends are eating this way so I can too". In just a few short years she is already seeing many positive changes in the way they think about food.

Laura also enjoys setting a great example of healthy lifestyle habits to her friends and loved ones. She's thrilled when one of them is interested in improving his/her lifestyle and she's right there to support that effort.

Her passion is to spread the word about the vast array of diet, exercise, and stress reduction information available. There are huge benefits to improving one's health instead of "waiting for something to break", then frantically trying to get better, or jumping into the trap of thinking a pill is going to fix the problem. She feels each day is a new opportunity to improve upon the day before. Never give up on yourself or your health!

Laura L Jackson RN
LauraRn@AHealthyApproach.com
www.AHealthyApproach.com

INDEX

15892689R00053

Made in the USA
Middletown, DE
26 November 2014